WHAT THE
Blues
IS ALL ABOUT

WHAT THE
Blues
IS ALL ABOUT

· · · · · · · · · ·

Black Women Overcoming
Stress and Depression

ANGELA MITCHELL

with Kennise Herring, Ph.D.

A PERIGEE BOOK

A Perigee Book
Published by The Berkley Publishing Group
A member of Penguin Putnam Inc.
200 Madison Avenue
New York, NY 10016

First edition: January 1998

Published simultaneously in Canada.

The Putnam Berkley World Wide Web site address is
http://www.berkley.com

Library of Congress Cataloging-in-Publication Data
Mitchell, Angela.
What the blues is all about : Black women overcoming stress and
depression / Angela Mitchell, with Kennise Herring.
    p.   cm.   "A Perigee book."
Includes bibliographical references (p. 235).
ISBN 0-399-52376-6
1. Depression, Mental—Popular works. 2. Afro-American women—
Mental health.   I. Title.
RC537.M563   1998
616.85'27'008996073—dc21   97-24482
                                CIP

Printed in the United States of America

2   4   6   8   10   9   7   5   3   1

To my mother, Gloria Elliott,
a woman of great courage.
Thank you for the gift
of your experience. —A.M.

Dedicated to the memory
of Kenneth Aubrey Herring,
who I now understand
suffered from an undiagnosed
mood disorder. —K.H.

Contents

Foreword   ix

Acknowledgments   xiii

Part I: What Is Depression?   1

Introduction: Tellin' It Like It Is: Seven Black Women
and Their Stories of Depression   3

1. What's Goin' On? Defining Depression
in Black Women   25

Part II: Stress and Depression in Black Women   49

2. The Mule of the World and Other Myths:
How Stereotypes of Black Women Contribute
to Depression   51

3. Living in the Integration Generation:
Race, Stress, and Depression   76

4. Love Don't Love Nobody: Self-Esteem, Relationships,
and Depression   94

5. Ain't Nobody's Business: Family Secrets, Shame, and Depression   111

6. Lay My Burden Down: Black Women and Suicide   128

Part III: Treatment, Self-Help, and Prevention   137

7. What Causes Depression?   139

8. There Is a Balm in Gilead: Finding Treatment for Depression   157

9. The Talking Cure: Psychotherapy for Depression   174

10. Drug Therapies and Other Treatments for Depression: The New Frontier?   192

11. Sisters Doin' It for Themselves: Self-Help and Prevention   214

12. Soul Serenade: Spirituality and Depression   224

13. Resources   231

Foreword

My friend John is a family practitioner. He often says that he has chosen the world's best profession. I disagree. I am a clinical psychologist, and though I rarely say it, I have chosen the world's greatest profession. I am afforded an opportunity to have an intimate, honest, confidential relationship with people that can profoundly affect both their lives and mine for the better. There are few things more fulfilling.

Whenever someone consults me for psychotherapy, I am acutely aware of how much courage it took to pick up the telephone and tell me that the pain of life is so great that something must be done. Walking into my office is probably the most difficult step many people take in their lives, and disclosing private matters that cause immense pain and disruption is simultaneously terrifying and relieving for those who see me. During their relationship with me, people learn a lot about themselves. This is to be expected, and I think and hope that the things my patients learn will help them create healthier and happier lives. I, too, learn an enormous amount about life, pain, joy, and myself. This was not something I expected when I selected the world's greatest profession, and it has been a wonderful surprise. The lessons my patients teach me have helped me grow in ways I never imagined, and I am sincerely grateful to them for contributing to my enrichment.

I have also learned that while the stigma about mental illness has lessened slightly over the past fifteen to twenty years, most people still feel embarrassed and ashamed at the thought of having a mental illness. People equate mental illnesses with weakness and character defects. Frequently, people feel that they should be able to get on with life in spite of debilitating emotional or psychological pain, such as the pain caused by depression. Somehow, for many people, being depressed is not the same as having physical illnesses. Consequently, many people quietly suffer for years with a treatable illness.

It is our hope that this book will provide you with some new information about an old illness. Perhaps you have been feeling sad for long periods of time, though everything seems fine on the surface. Maybe you know someone who is moody and irritable; she never seems to feel that anything is going well and you hate being around her. You and your friends think she has a bad attitude. After reading this book, you may learn that she has little if any control over her moods. From your perspective, things may be going well for her, but her perception and experience of life is radically different. She feels like there is a dark cloud over her head on the clearest and sunniest of days. She spends each waking moment in agony. If this book can help you understand her and help her get the care she needs, then we have achieved our goal. We want to help people recognize and treat depression.

Though depression is common in all women, we have written this book specifically for Black women. Studies have found (and we know from experience) that African Americans tend to be less informed about mental illness, and as a result, often fail to get the appropriate treatment. We also know that many African Americans are wary of psychologists, social workers, and other mental health practitioners. We believe we can make a useful contribution by offering some basic factual information about mental health, psychotherapy, medications, Black women, and depression.

The book is written in three parts. In part one, we give voice to seven valiant women who have lived with depression. We are immensely grateful to these women for taking the time to talk to us about their private pain. These women are not our patients, and it was extremely kind and generous of them to help us try to help others.

In part two, we talk about how the blues are different from depression. We discuss the denigrating myths and stereotypes about Black women that we think contribute to both becoming depressed and to the difficulties we have in getting treatment for depression. We also talk about stress, self-esteem, family secrets, and shame. In part three, we introduce theories of depressive illness, treatment, self-help, and prevention. We have offered a few resources that we hope you will find useful.

To paraphrase Marvin Gaye, there are far too many of us crying. It is our sincere hope that this book will help put an end to the tears.

—K.H.

Acknowledgments

In the six years that I have lived with this book, I have learned a tremendous amount about depression and our ability to overcome it. I have also learned how generous and open people can be, even with the most difficult and personal information. The women we interviewed for this project all expressed a desire to help others suffering from depression by sharing their own stories. I am extremely grateful for their willingness to participate in this process. Without them, there would be no book.

I have been blessed to find such a knowledgeable, professional, and perceptive collaborator in Kennise Herring. Her diligent work on this project has been a lifesaver. Only our personal relationship means more to me than our professional one. I must also thank Hubert, Franklin, Victoria, and Samuel for allowing me to take up so much of her time.

Denise Stinson has seen this book through from beginning to end, and there is no doubt in my mind that she is largely responsible for its existence. She was able to help me find the book in my jumble of ideas. Suzanne Bober's insightful editing and great patience are also very much appreciated.

Thank you, thank you to my friend and mentor, Thulani Davis, who has taught me much of what I know about writing and even more of what I know about life. In conversations over the kitchen table and across long-distance phone lines, she, Dawn Crossland, and Deborah Thomas have contributed more to this effort than I can articulate. Thanks also to Beth Davis for many long, thought-provoking conversations about life as a Black woman, and to Teresa Wiltz for prodding me (gently and with empathy) when I procrastinated.

Thank you to the Henry J. Kaiser Family Foundation for giving me the time and freedom to explore this idea, and especially to Penny Duckham and the class of '94 for sharing your expertise with me.

Finally, thanks to Rogers Mitchell and Gloria Elliott for encouraging (and being proud of) me and my writing, and to my wonderful husband, Craig Nakamoto, for being my shelter in the storm.

—*Angela Mitchell*

I want to thank Angela Mitchell for allowing me to have an opportunity to work on this wonderful project. What began as an inquiring telephone call has developed into a warm, respectful, intimate friendship that I am certain will continue long after this project. I also want to thank Juanita F. Herring and Hubert O. Thompson for a belief in me that has been more important than I can ever articulate. You were inspirational in my writing about depression many years ago. Thank you!

Finally, thank you to Franklin, Victoria, and Samuel for being so patient with me all of those times I sat at the computer and didn't let you type.

—*Kennise Herring, Ph.D.*

WHAT THE
Blues
IS ALL ABOUT

PART I

· · · · · · · · · ·

WHAT IS
DEPRESSION?

Introduction

Tellin' It Like It Is:
Seven Black Women and
Their Stories of Depression

"I hate Mondays. They depress me."

"My man and I broke up last night, and I'm really depressed about it."

"I can't watch the news anymore. It's too depressing."

Depressed. It's a word we use often, whenever something makes us feel down. We say we are depressed when things don't go the way we want them to—when we lose a job or a lover, when money troubles keep creditors calling, when it rains for two weeks straight. We use the word *depressed* to describe a mood—when you're depressed, you're blue, you're in a sad place. By these definitions, depression is an everyday occurrence. It is what we feel when we're in the valleys of life, when we're wandering in the wilderness.

Everyone feels depressed at some point in time. Feelings of depression are a normal and healthy response to loss and disappointment. We expect to feel sad when a loved one dies or after a divorce. In fact, we'd probably worry about someone who didn't feel sad or depressed under such circumstances.

But not all depressions are the same. Sometimes depression is more than feeling sad, more than having the blues. Depression can be a long-term—even lifelong—war with profound feelings of hopelessness and low self-esteem. Sometimes it is a daily struggle to get out of bed, to go to work, and to do what you need to do.

Depression can be lethal. Mental health professionals have termed this kind of depression *major depression* or *clinical depression.* Clinical depression takes over the mind and makes you feel as if you will never see light again. It can last for weeks or months and recur for years, smothering your life, sapping your strength, and perhaps stealing your desire to live. It is dangerous; about 15 percent of all clinically depressed people eventually commit suicide. It costs millions of dollars in lost productivity each year, and the costs to relationships and self-esteem can't be quantified. As many as 9 percent of American women are depressed at any given time, and 20 to 25 percent will become depressed at some point in their lives. (Women are twice as likely as men to suffer from depression—only 3 percent of American men are depressed at any given time; up to 12 percent will become depressed during their lifetimes.) There are no statistics on the rate of depression in African Americans (men or women), but researchers assume, based on limited studies, that the rate of depression in Blacks is about the same as that of whites.

Fortunately, there are successful treatments—as many as 80 percent of people who are treated for depression do get better. But Black women rarely receive the proper diagnosis or treatment. By some estimates, only 7 percent of Black women suffering from depression receive any treatment, compared to 20 percent of the general population. Why? The possible explanations are familiar: we are misdiagnosed by doctors, we don't recognize the symptoms, we don't know treatment exists, and we don't demand it. Many times, depressed African Americans go to their primary-care doctors or to hospital emergency rooms for help with their symptoms. However, even though depression is extremely common, only one-third to one-half of the cases are actually recognized by primary-care doctors. Another explanation might be that many of us find it hard to fathom that we are depressed. Accepting the diagnosis of depression (or any other mental illness) can be very difficult. Renee, one of the women interviewed for this book, seemed to have both these problems. Though the first doctor she saw in a hospital emergency room did recognize that she was depressed, Renee could not accept the diagnosis. She then went back and forth to the emergency room and various doctors for nine years, and none of these doctors correctly diagnosed her depression.

Much of the suffering caused by depression can be stopped. The first step to reducing the effects of depression on our lives is recognizing it in ourselves and those we love. Then we must make sure psychiatrists, psychologists, and others who diagnose and treat depression recognize our symptoms as well. We must also try to understand it: What causes depression? Are the causes or symptoms any different in Black women? Finally, our depression must be treated. We must educate ourselves about the available treatments, dispel the myths about treatment, and overcome our fears of medication and psychotherapy. We must become advocates for ourselves and those close to us. This book is the first step toward helping Black women find their way out of the darkness of depression.

Am I Depressed?
Will This Book Help Me?

Maybe you're wondering if you are or someone close to you is depressed. Or perhaps your doctor has told you that you are depressed, but you don't know what to do about it. This book can help you determine if what you've been feeling is depression and help guide you after the diagnosis is made. It will answer questions like:

- Why am I always crying?
- Why can't I eat or sleep?
- How is depression different from the blues?
- What causes depression?
- Is depression psychological or biological?
- What is the best treatment for depression?
- Will I have to take medication for the rest of my life?
- What happens in psychotherapy?
- Is God trying to punish me?

If you have pondered these kinds of questions, keep reading.

Seven Sisters' Stories of Depression

Throughout this book, you will hear the voices of seven Black women living with clinical depression. These women are young and not-so-young. They are overworked and unemployed; single, married, and divorced; gay and straight. Some have had moderate, passing bouts of depression; others have struggled with severe depressive episodes for most of their lives. All of them know what it is like to completely lose hope, and all have managed to find it again.

Listen as these seven sisters tell their stories. Perhaps you will see yourself—or someone you love—in them.

Celeste

Celeste, a forty-year-old health-policy analyst, was diagnosed with major depressive disorder five years ago. Looking back, Celeste now thinks she first became depressed while she was in her teens. She struggled with mild to moderate bouts of depression throughout her twenties and thirties, but didn't seek treatment until she suffered her most serious depressive episode at thirty-five.

At that time, Celeste was under tremendous stress. She had

WHAT WE THINK ABOUT DEPRESSION

A 1996 survey conducted by the National Mental Health Association found that African Americans are confused about the definition, causes, and symptoms of depression.

- Sixty-three percent of us think depression is a personal weakness. **Depression is not a personal weakness; it is a treatable mental illness.**
- Only 31 percent of us think depression is a health problem. **Depression and other mental disorders *are* health problems.**
- Fifty-nine percent of us think it is normal for a woman to be depressed during menopause.
- Fifty-six percent think depression is a normal part of aging. **Depression is not normal at any stage of life.**
- Forty-five percent believe it is normal for a mother to feel depressed for at least two weeks after having a baby. **Many new mothers may experience a few days of baby blues after giving birth, but depression that lasts for two weeks or more is not a normal part of childbirth.**
- Forty percent believe it is normal for a husband or wife to feel depressed for more than a year after the death of their spouse. **Feeling lonely, lost, and sad is a part of the grieving process. But depression that lasts more than six months after the loss of a loved one is not normal.**

Myths like these keep us from recognizing depression and getting the treatment we need. They make it hard for us to support our loved ones who are suffering from depression or to ask for help when we need it. Depression is common, but it is not normal. No one wants to be depressed, and no one should have to just live with it.

just started a new job at a major foundation—a job she wasn't even sure she wanted. Celeste had been happy at her previous job, but she was recruited heavily, "wined and dined" as she describes it, by the foundation. She weighed her options carefully and asked everyone she knew for advice. She came to the conclusion that even though she was satisfied with her job at the time, she would want to move up within the next year or so. Why not now?

The first few months at the foundation were wonderful: Celeste got to pursue her own interests and work independently, two things that were very important to her. Just as she was settling in, the program director in her area, who had encouraged Celeste's interests, was fired. The new program director had a totally different vision for the department—and for Celeste's position. Over the next few months, Celeste became more and more disenchanted. "Everything that had been promised in this job evaporated," Celeste says. "I was doing exactly the job I feared I would be doing." So she dealt with her disappointment the way she always did: by throwing herself into her work. She knew she was unhappy, but the more unhappy she became, the more industrious she was. "I was just this superachiever, which made me get tireder and tireder," she remembers. "And I was more frustrated that the job still wasn't what I wanted. I really started to go down."

Celeste wasn't getting any relief on the home front, either. Jason, her husband of ten years, had just quit his job on a whim and was making no effort to help foot the bills. They had recently bought a house, and the mortgage had to be paid. Celeste now had to bear that responsibility herself. She also single-handedly cared for their eight-year-old twin sons, who were having a lot of trouble in school at the time. To top it all off, Celeste got no emotional support from Jason. She would soon learn that he was having an affair.

Celeste felt her world slipping away from her. She knew a little about depression, and began to suspect that it was happening to her. "I was very tired and very sad," she remembers. "I felt hopeless, and eventually, I started feeling suicidal. . . . I'd drive home from work and I would argue with myself about why I shouldn't hit the barricade, why I shouldn't just run into something. Or when a train was coming, why I shouldn't jump in front of it," Celeste remembers. "My well had run dry. There was nothing left. On the weekends, I couldn't even get out of bed."

Celeste had the classic symptoms of major depression. She was sad and hopeless, and even though she was able to continue working, she found no pleasure in it. She managed to drag herself through her workdays, but was so fatigued when the weekend came that she could barely move. She began to blame herself for her pain: she believed that all her choices had been bad ones. She shouldn't have taken the new job, she shouldn't have married her husband, she shouldn't have had the children. Celeste started seeing a psychiatrist for psychotherapy when she first became depressed, and he prescibed antidepressants. They were not effective, however, and now Celeste was actively suicidal. She had devised a plan to park her car in a garage and take an overdose of antidepressant pills. She had even written a suicide note.

Celeste had managed to keep her depression a secret until she was hospitalized. She tried to keep on keepin' on. "When I'm at my worst, I look my best," she explains. "I don't let it show. I don't want people to know I'm having problems. I'm ashamed and embarrassed." And when friends and family members did learn of her depression, most of them did not understand it. "People would give me suggestions like 'Well, get up and do something.' I'd try to 'do something' and it wouldn't work. I would try to read. Nothing worked."

Celeste spent two weeks on the psychiatric unit, and, following her discharge, entered a day-treatment program (where she spent days at the hospital but went home at night) for two more weeks. The treatment process has been difficult, however. She has not responded well to most of the medications she has tried. Celeste is trying to cope with her depression day by day. Her work with her therapist has helped Celeste better understand her depression and put her life experiences in perspective. She is thankful for that. But Celeste is still in the process of recovery, and she realizes her journey toward wellness will probably be lifelong.

Keisha

Like Celeste, Keisha first became depressed in her teens. She remembers writing "I wish I were dead" in her diary as a thirteen-year-old junior-high student. She is now twenty-three, but in some ways feels as if she has already lived a lifetime. Keisha has been diagnosed with a major depressive disorder with psychotic features.

On the surface, there is nothing about Keisha's life that would make you think she would be haunted by such severe depressions. She grew up in an upper-middle-class suburb, the youngest of three children. Her parents, who have been married for over thirty years, were very involved in their children's lives and always encouraged them to strive for the best. Keisha and her siblings all excelled academically, from elementary school through college. Her family seemed to live an enchanted life.

The enchantment ended abruptly when one summer evening, a year after finishing college, Keisha tried to take her life. She had been depressed since a few months after graduating from college—jobs were hard to come by that year, and Keisha was extremely discouraged. She was also having trouble adjusting to living at home after four years of being on her own. A few weeks before the suicide attempt that sent her to the hospital, Keisha rigged a noose in her basement and planned to hang herself. Every night, after her parents had gone to bed, Keisha would go to the basement, stand on a chair, and put her head in the noose. Fortunately, she never could bring herself to commit suicide in this way (suicide attempts by hanging are almost always successful).

Keisha's suicidal feelings did not go away. One night, her parents went out. She drank a bottle of wine and took three bottles of pills—one of which was the antidepressant she had been prescribed. Right before she blacked out, Keisha called her next door neighbors and told them what she had done. They immediately called an ambulance. Keisha doesn't know what made her call the neighbors. "It was almost like I was on automatic pilot and someone else took over my body. I really don't remember doing it," she says.

Keisha had a history of serious depressions before this suicide attempt. She remembers being very withdrawn, sad, and lonely in junior high, around the time she made the diary entry. But her first truly severe depression occurred right before she left home for college. A breakup with a boyfriend triggered the episode, which left Keisha with familiar feelings of loneliness and sadness, and a strong sense of wanting to end it all. She thought she had no support. "I felt that all my friends were rejecting me, that they didn't care about me anymore," she remembers. "All my friends had boyfriends and they spent all their time with them. They didn't seem to have time for me. I was really hurt by that." She also felt worthless. "I had really low self-esteem; I didn't think much of myself," she admits. Keisha began to have fleeting thoughts of suicide. "Once I was in a car and I wanted to see what would happen if I just turned off the road," she says.

Keisha began seeing a psychologist for psychotherapy that summer, and she entered college in the fall as planned. The excitement of college seemed to do her good: She made it through that semester without becoming depressed. But the loneliness returned with winter, and she began to see a therapist at school. She felt better after a few months, and stopped the therapy when school let out again in June.

Keisha continued on this kind of roller coaster for the next few years. Breakups seemed to trigger many of her depressive episodes, and each episode was worse than the last. She also began having panic attacks. A psychiatrist prescribed antidepressant and antianxiety medication for her, but her depressions became more and more frightening. She lost her appetite and shed eighteen pounds in a few weeks. She couldn't sleep through the night. She cried incessantly. Keisha began to drink heavily, and finally, on that summer evening, she decided she'd had enough.

After that suicide attempt, Keisha was hospitalized on the psychiatric unit for several weeks and then spent several more weeks in a day-treatment program. She remained on antidepressant and antianxiety medication and stayed in therapy. Over time, she began to feel better. But a year later, Keisha again attempted suicide. Her psychiatrist determined that Keisha had symptoms of a thought disorder when depressed (her thoughts were racing and disjointed), and started her on an antipsychotic medication in addition to the antidepressant and antianxiety medications.

Keisha is trying to regain control over her life. She moved in with her parents again after the second suicide attempt, and although she feels a little safer there, she says she is still apprehensive. "I am just scared of when the next episode is going to come," Keisha admits. She is planning to attend graduate school soon, and is working on getting her self-confidence back. "In general, I feel hopeful about the future . . . but I wonder how things would be different if I didn't have depression," she muses. Keisha also wishes more people understood depression. "I've had my mom say to me, 'You just need to stop thinking about yourself all the time.' If I could stop, I would. Why would I want to hate myself?"

Latrice
When we asked twenty-five-year-old Latrice about her hopes for the future, she laughed softly and said, "I hope the next

twenty-five years are nothing like the first twenty-five." We understood what she meant.

Latrice doesn't know how long she has been having "mood swings"—her name for her depressive episodes. She remembers feeling depressed as a teenager, but she thinks the episodes actually started when she was a little girl. The most recent one came after Latrice got into a car accident and ended up in jail overnight. She had been driving on a suspended license—she had several tickets and couldn't afford to pay them—and her insurance had been canceled because she couldn't afford to pay that, either. When she failed to show up in court on a speeding ticket, she was arrested. Finding herself in jail, she "freaked out." "I was crying and hyperventilating," she remembers. "They threw me in a cell. They took all my clothes and they gave me this paper gown to wear. And I was sitting there thinking, *This cannot be an episode in my life.* But it was."

Latrice was upset with herself for letting things get so out of hand. She refused to let anyone bail her out, especially her eighty-eight-year-old grandfather, who had bailed her out of messes so many times. So she stayed in jail overnight, plotting how she was going to dig her way out of the hole she was in. The more she plotted, the deeper the hole seemed. By the time she got out of jail the next day, she felt even worse. She needed her car to get to work, but she didn't have enough money to get it out of the auto pound (it had been impounded after the accident). Nor did she have enough money to pay the outstanding tickets or her auto insurance. She had no hope of making money if she didn't have a car, but she couldn't get the car without money. And she felt she couldn't ask the one person who would give her the money—her grandfather. She became even more depressed. There seemed to be no way out. Latrice began the familiar ritual of staying in her room, crying, and eating.

Luckily, Latrice did have some support. She had been seeing

a therapist for several months, since her last depressive episode. That episode was more serious, and though she is not sure about what in her own life triggered it, she does remember it starting right around the time singer Phyllis Hyman committed suicide. "I can understand why she [Hyman] killed herself," Latrice explains. "Sometimes you get so sad, and you don't know how not to be sad. It's like the only thing to stop the sadness is to die." This "mood swing" seemed to envelop Latrice one night as she sat in bed watching television. She suddenly felt the urge to pull the car into the garage, close the door, and run the engine. A few days later, while on a boat with some friends, she again felt a suicidal impulse, this time telling her to jump. And one day, while walking on an elevated concourse in a high-rise building, she thought, "If I went up there and jumped, would I just really injure myself or would I kill myself?" Latrice told her therapist about these suicidal thoughts, and was referred to a psychiatrist who prescribed the antidepressant Paxil for her. But Latrice never filled the prescription. "I couldn't afford it," she says.

Where did all this sadness come from? In Latrice's case, the sadness, hopelessness, and low self-esteem have been building since her early childhood. She has survived horrible physical, emotional, and sexual abuse. And like many, if not most, abuse survivors, she is chronically depressed. She seems to have *double depression*: dysthymia (a mild, chronic depression) interrupted by periods of major depression. Some days she makes it through OK; many days she is overcome by crying spells that seem to come out of nowhere. Some days she wants to end her life.

Latrice has dreams of becoming a singer, but right now she is still trying to find her voice—the voice that can speak about the betrayal and abuse she suffered. With the help of her therapist, Latrice is working through her intense anger and her depression. She has vowed to do everything in her power to insure that her next twenty-five years are nothing like the first twenty-five.

Elaine

Although she'd had many hard times in her life, Elaine didn't have a true depressive episode until she was sixty-four years old. She describes how, bit by bit, her life unraveled. It started with her increasing irritability. Elaine had always been very upbeat and cheerful, so much so that her family nicknamed her Merry Sunshine. But beginning in the winter of her sixty-fourth year, she started to feel on edge and testy, not like herself at all. She became short-tempered at work, which caused friction with her coworkers. It didn't help that she was caught in the midst of a power struggle at the school where she taught. Elaine got so fed up that she retired abruptly, unceremoniously ending a stellar twenty-five-year teaching career. Then, without a job, she became overwhelmed by financial worries. She started to regret her decision to retire, then she picked apart every major decision she had made in her life, concluding that all of them had been miserably wrong. She was a failure at everything she had done. She was too embarrassed to tell anyone how she felt, so she stopped talking to her friends. She instructed her daughter, Nona, to tell anyone who called that she was out of town.

Soon, Elaine couldn't get out of bed. "I literally could not get my legs over the edge of the bed," she recalls. She would lie in darkness all day, wringing her hands and worrying. She saw no hope of anything ever changing, and no way out of her misery. A devout Catholic, Elaine did talk to a priest when she first started to feel suicidal. He took her to the hospital, where she was admitted to the psychiatric unit, given antidepressants, and was discharged a few days later. The despondency returned within a week. She took an overdose of her antidepressant medication and was hospitalized for six weeks.

Over the next two years, Elaine suffered increasingly debilitating bouts of depression. A little over a year after her release from the hospital after her first suicide attempt, she made her most serious attempt. She again took an overdose of her medication, but this time followed it up with a large amount of whiskey. She then drove herself to a secluded forest preserve and sat alone under a tree, waiting to die. It is only because of the concern of a stranger that she is alive today. She stumbled upon a family having a picnic, and one of them took her to the hospital.

Thankfully, Elaine did survive, and she finally received the treatment that she needed. She spent nine months in a day-hospital program, where she participated in group therapy and other activities that helped her come out of her depression. Even so, she didn't understand that her depression was a chronic illness, and that she would have to be on antidepressant medication for the rest of her life. When she stopped taking the medication after deciding that she felt better and didn't need it, she became depressed and ended up in the hospital again.

Four years after her first encounter with major depression, Elaine has begun to come to terms with the chronic nature of her illness. She takes her medication every day now, without fail, knowing what will happen if she doesn't. Elaine can talk about her depression now. She realizes that she shouldn't be ashamed of it. "I have an illness," she says. "That's all."

Nona

Nona is Elaine's thirty-year-old daughter. It has taken her a long time to realize that she, too, suffers from depression, though when she really thinks about it, she believes that it started when she was very young.

Growing up, Nona was a daddy's girl. Though her father drank heavily until Nona was seven years old (he quit after being told he would die within a year if he continued), she spent much of her time with him, puttering around in the garage, working on science projects, and just sitting in his lap, daydreaming. It was no secret that Nona loved her father.

Nona's parents divorced when she was thirteen, and she now thinks she first became depressed soon thereafter. Although she expected the divorce, she was devastated when her father moved out. Years later, Nona finds it hard to distinguish between what might have been depression and what were just the effects of puberty, but she does recall wanting to die, and saying so. "I would scream 'I wish I was never born' to my mother, and that would just send her off. I don't think she ever thought I meant it."

Nona and her mother fought a great deal during this time, and Nona sometimes became violent. "Once I got so angry that I punched a hole in my bedroom wall. Another time I threw my phone at the wall. I would throw coffee cups and glasses across the room in the middle of an argument. The worst time was when I almost slammed my mother's arm in the bathroom door." Surprisingly, neither Nona nor her mother recognized that she was out of control. They both thought this was normal adolescent behavior. Nona's mother did threaten to send her to live with her father a few times, but she never followed through.

After about a year, things seemed to settle down. Nona and her mother started to get along very well. And Nona looked forward to going away to college. When she was accepted at an East Coast school, Nona jumped at the chance to broaden her horizons.

At first, college was great. No parents, no rules, no classes she didn't want to take. But after a fight with her roommate (who had been her best friend since ninth grade), something changed. Nona and her roommate stopped talking. She felt like she had lost a sister. Nona started having trouble studying. She began to think she wasn't smart enough to make it at the competitive college she attended. She somehow managed to pull through her first semester.

The second semester was a different story. Nona was doing poorly in her classes. Again, she had trouble concentrating. Her papers were late; she couldn't focus enough to study for her exams. By the time finals came around, she was overcome with fear. She stayed in her room for three days, barely eating or sleeping, until friends urged her to see the school psychologist. She did, and he determined that she was in no shape to take her exams. She went home that summer and tried to forget how hard the year had been.

Sophomore year brought another episode. This time, a breakup with a boyfriend sent her spiraling down. Nona's mother came to visit one weekend and found her daughter unusually reserved and distant. Over brunch, Nona told her mother that she "felt like the unluckiest person in the world," though, objectively, things were going very well for her. Nona's mother, concerned and angry, told Nona she didn't ever want to hear her say such a thing again. "She told me I was blessed, how dare I say I was unlucky," Nona recalls. "But that's how I felt. I know it may not have been rational, but I truly felt as if everything that could go wrong, had gone wrong. I had screwed up my first year of school; my boyfriend dumped me and then wouldn't even talk to me when he saw me on campus. I felt ugly, unpopular, unable to do well academically, and unlucky. But I think telling my mother that made her angry because she was working very hard to keep me in school, to pay my tuition. To sacrifice for your daughter and then hear her say, essentially, 'This means nothing to me,' I think that made her really angry."

Throughout her college years, Nona was plagued with episodes like this. Though her girlfriends recognized that something was wrong, they weren't sure what the problem might be. At one point, a close friend got so concerned that she called Nona's mother, who tried to convince her daughter to see the school psychologist again. Nona refused. "I thought I could handle it by myself," she says. "I felt that I knew myself well. I didn't need some stranger analyzing me." Instead, Nona began to drink. A bad day often meant a bottle of Jack Daniel's. Frustrated and confused, some of Nona's friends began to pull away.

Even so, Nona would not get help.

After a while, Nona's ups and downs seemed to become part of her personality. No one thought much of them until she hit a new low in her mid-twenties. After the man she was dating (and in love with) told her he was not in love with her, Nona felt as if the ground had collapsed beneath her. She cried for hours every night. She could barely get herself to work, and she cried all day once she was there. One day, wanting to die, she inched herself out of the bathroom window on the twelfth floor of the building where she worked. Terrified by what she was thinking, she came in. A few nights later, she dissolved a box of over-the-counter sleeping pills into a cup of water and took a sip. But she couldn't go through with it, and she called her by then ex-boyfriend, who talked to her until she calmed down. The next day, a friend at work suggested that psychotherapy might help her. She agreed.

Therapy was a great help to Nona, though her therapist never actually told her she was depressed. Nona didn't realize that she might have been depressed until her mother became ill about a year later. She continued in therapy, off and on, for several years, however, and credits it with keeping her moderate depressive episodes from becoming more severe.

Now married, Nona still has periods of depression. The worst came when she was taking birth control pills. She had gotten used to taking to her bed, immobile and weepy, for several days each month. But her husband thought something was wrong and suggested that she stop taking the pills. Since then, Nona's depressive episodes have become more infrequent.

Nona wonders what the future will bring. "I guess I have to

admit that depression runs in my family,'' she says. ''I just hope that we can stop it here.''

Renee

Renee, thirty-three, has also been depressed since her teens, but she wasn't diagnosed until she was twenty-one. She was convinced early on that there was something wrong with her, but she never thought the problem might be depression. Renee had been experiencing a number of physical symptoms since high school. She frequently had headaches so severe that they blurred her vision. Once she had chest pains and thought she was having a heart attack. She felt sad and tired, too, but the possibility that she might have a mental illness never crossed her mind. Writing seemed to be the only thing that helped her through these terrifying episodes. She wrote this while in the depths of one of her depressions:

> All I can do is to write while I am in bed. When the out of control feeling comes, I head for the bed. Sometimes I can fight it, and most times I do. My mother just asked me, "What kind of pain is it?" I'm going to try to explain. When it's hard, it feels like the life is being drawn out of me. First I become weak and it seems like I lose my brain or like I'm moving my limbs—like I'm moving in slow motion. I feel like I'm falling, but I fight it. My blood feels like it's boiling and it's having a hard time getting through the vessels, my head pounds and feels like a numbing sensation. I have a hard time swallowing when it is really bad, and I have a shaky feeling. When it's not bad, I still have a shaky feeling without the other symptoms.

During one particularly bad depressive episode, Renee's mother and grandmother became quite worried. ''I was very sick; I couldn't get up,'' Renee remembers. ''I was very tired; I had no energy; I was crying a lot. I think I was in the bed for about a week." Frightened, Renee's grandmother took her to a hospital emergency room, where a doctor diagnosed her with major depression. "I thought, *Oh, no.* I didn't believe it. I couldn't believe that this was a mental problem." But Renee felt so horrible that she took the medication anyway, hoping it would bring some relief. Soon, most of her symptoms subsided and she stopped taking the antidepressant, though she still felt "not quite right." About two months later, she felt the depression returning. "I was very tired again," Renee recalls. "I couldn't concentrate enough to get any of my schoolwork done. I would have to take days off from school. And I felt very sad." Renee went to a different doctor. But this time, she got no answers.

Over the next nine years, still not believing that she had a mental illness, Renee went from doctor to doctor, trying to find out what was wrong with her. Many of those visits were to the same county hospital clinic. But despite very clear depressive symptoms—sadness, lethargy, feeling weighted down, bodily aches and pains—no one realized that she was depressed. "I thought I had a brain tumor or something," she says. Doctors gave her every test imaginable, for everything from gynecological to glandular problems. No one diagnosed the obvious. And Renee still wasn't ready to accept that she was, in fact, depressed.

Finally, just three years ago, one doctor suggested that Renee see a psychiatrist. "I didn't want to go," she says. "I thought seeing a psychiatrist would mean I was crazy, that I was losing control. But I had been praying about it, and I thought God was telling me that this was what I should do. So I decided to go."

Three months after that recommendation, Renee made an appointment with a psychiatrist. He told her the same thing that she had learned on her first visit to the emergency room nine years earlier: she had major depression. He prescribed another antidepressant, Zoloft, which made Renee sick to her stomach, and then switched her to the same one she had taken originally, Norprimin. Again, it seemed to work for her. This time she stayed on it.

Although the medication did alleviate the tiredness and other physical symptoms Renee felt, there was one feeling she just couldn't shake. "Even though I go about my life, there is this deep sadness," she says. This inescapable sadness recently led her to a psychologist for psychotherapy. Renee is hopeful that her work in therapy will help her understand the source of her pain (which is undoubtedly related, at least in part, to the fact that she has lost four siblings and an uncle to whom she was very close), and, ultimately, overcome it.

Maya

Maya, thirty-eight, has also been battling depression since her teens. Unlike most of the women we interviewed, however, Maya does not have major depression. Maya suffers from dysthymia, a milder, chronic depressive illness. While she has never felt so desperate that she tried to take her life, she can't recall ever feeling really good for an extended period of time, either. "I guess I had episodes of happiness as a child," she says. "But I never felt basically happy. I always felt like there was some sort of conflict going on inside of me."

Maya remembers first noticing that she was depressed soon after her beloved grandfather died. She was fifteen at the time. "I recognized that this feeling I had was something more than just the blues," she says. "It seemed to last longer. It was deeper, it felt more profound, and it was something specific. I remember crying an awful lot and hiding in dark rooms a lot. I wanted to be by myself as much as possible. I didn't eat very much—it was like my appetite just wasn't there."

While Maya remembers that her family did acknowledge that she was depressed at this time, they didn't think anything of it. After all, her grandfather had just passed away. She had good reason to be depressed. What they didn't realize was that

Maya never seemed really happy, even before her grandfather's death. They just assumed her quiet, withdrawn demeanor was a personality trait. They didn't know—or at least they didn't let on that they knew—the secrets Maya was keeping. Maya had been sexually abused by her aunt, who lived in the same building, for years. She was also watching her mother slowly kill herself with alcohol. And to complicate matters further, Maya had begun to realize that she was gay.

"Over time, the grief that I felt that contributed to the depression started to lessen," Maya says. "I also became more involved with academics, and then I started getting into what I felt was a very dangerous but exciting hidden life around discovering that I was lesbian."

Though many gay teens find the process of discovering and exploring their sexuality traumatic, it was liberating for Maya. She had been dating boys for a few years and always felt as if something were missing. Now she knew why, and she had a new world—and a new self—to discover. She believes that discovering her sexuality helped her come out of her depression. "It focused my mind on something else that was outside of me," she says. "It wasn't about me strictly. It was about this whole big life experience." Even so, this was a frightening time for Maya. "I was in a lot of turmoil," she remembers. "I was scared because I felt like I was doing this on my own. At that time I didn't have friends that I thought I could talk to about [being a lesbian]."

Maya was also having trouble with her mother during this time. "I had been having huge conflicts with my mother over where I was going to go to school." Maya attended the neighborhood high school, which was known more for the drug dealing that went on there than for educating its students. She had an opportunity to attend an honors program at another school, farther away from home, but her mother wouldn't let her. To make matters worse, Maya's mother became very ill, suffering a series of congestive heart failures in a short span of time.

"We went through all of that at the same time," recalls Maya. "I didn't feel supported about school, and I didn't know that there was anybody out there that I could discuss all these transitions with." Her depressive feelings ebbed and flowed throughout this time, and worsened when, about a year later, her mother died. That was the only time she actually felt suicidal, though the feeling soon passed. She found a therapist—a clinical social worker at a youth services agency—and feels that therapy has been her lifeline.

To this day, Maya still isn't sure she's ever felt truly happy. She has spent years in the same job, frustrated with the racism that contributes to her lack of advancement. She feels stuck— in the city she grew up in, which she would like to leave; in the job she hates; and in her dysthymia. She and her therapist are working on getting her unstuck, but that process is a slow and deliberate one.

Without question, each of these women has endured incredible pain. Yet, the fact that they talked so openly about their depression is evidence that each one is currently winning the battle with this baffling illness. Peace of mind has not come easily for any of these women, but it has come, even if only in glimpses. These glimpses offer a hope that has kept these women alive and has led them into treatment. Perhaps their hope will inspire you to hope, as well.

1

· · · · · · ·

What's Goin' On? Defining
Depression in Black Women

Depressive Illness and the Mood Disorders:
An Introduction

The word *depression* is commonly used to describe what might be better termed *the depressions*. Depression is not one disorder. There are several types, ranging from mild dysthymia to severe, recurrent, major depression. Some types of depression are thought to be principally biological in origin, and others are thought to be more situational or psychological. Some depressions seem to readily lend themselves to treatment with antidepressant drugs, and others respond equally well to psychotherapy. This diversity of depressions has bred much confusion and disagreement among those who study and treat the disorder, and this confusion can make life for those living with depression even more trying than it already is.

Those who study and treat depression have tried to eliminate some of this confusion by establishing a system to determine whether or not a person is depressed, and if she is, what type of depression she seems to have. This diagnostic system, set forth in the American Psychiatric Association's *Diagnostic and Statistical Manual of Mental Disorders, Fourth Edition* (DSM-IV), is the generally accepted means of diagnosing depression (and all other mental and emotional disorders). The system is not without its flaws, however, and there are those who choose to ignore DSM-IVs classifications altogether. Nevertheless, the DSM-IV is the most commonly accepted means of diagnosing mental illness and emotional disorders, and its definition is the one we will use in our discussion of depression.

In the DSM-IV, the depressions fall under an umbrella of illnesses called *mood disorders*. As the name implies, disturbances in mood (sadness, apathy, anxiety, excitability, and irritability) are the main feature of mood disorders. These disturbances are not the familiar feelings associated with everyday moodiness. These mood disorders cause profound suffering and lead people to behave in ways they wouldn't ordinarily. Furthermore, although mood disturbances are the most obvious symptoms of mood disorders, they are only part of the picture. Mood disorders are comprised of a variety of symptoms that affect most aspects of a person's life: emotions, thoughts, behavior, even the way a person feels physically.

There are two main types of mood disorders: *Depressive* (or *unipolar*) disorders and *bipolar* disorders. The depressive disorders include major depression (also called *clinical depression* or *unipolar depression*); *dysthymia* (a milder, chronic form of depression); and a catchall category called depressive disorder not otherwise specified, which includes minor and brief depressions and those associated with seasonal changes and the menstrual cycle. Bipolar disorders include what is commonly called *manic-depression* and *cyclothymia* (a milder, chronic form of bipolar disorder).

The Depressive Disorders

Each of the depressive disorders is distinct from the others, but they all have one thing in common: depressed mood. At some point, all people diagnosed with depressive disorders feel tremendously sad. They often describe feeling numb. They may be weepy and full of worries, or they may withdraw and become completely disconnected from the world. No efforts to cheer them up seem to make any difference.

Two things distinguish one depressive disorder from another: severity and duration. Major depression is the most severe depressive disorder, while dysthymia is less severe but lasts much longer. Other depressive disorders vary in severity and last anywhere from a few days to a lifetime. We hear the most about major depression, probably because it is both the most common and the most debilitating of the depressions. It is also the form of depression that most often leads to tragedy. The suicides of vibrant Black women like singer Phyllis Hyman, journalist Leanita McClain, and writer Terri Jewell remind us that major depression can be a killer. In this case, however, knowledge and proper treatment can stop this killer.

Major Depression

I was sitting in my bed watching TV. And all of a sudden, it felt like I had a black wave come up from behind. I just had this crying spell. . . . It came out of nowhere; it didn't mean anything, it was nothing specific that I was doing. Earlier that day, I was on the phone talkin' and trippin' out with my friends. And then later I'm sittin' in the room and all of a sudden I just felt this blackness. All of a sudden, I felt out of control. I told myself, "Okay, well, I'm going to calm down, calm down." The more I tried to calm down, the more upset I got. At that point, I was like, "I'm going to pull the car into the garage and I'm going to run the engine. That'll do it." It got beyond me. It's not something that I would want to do, it's just something I was thinking about doing. And I couldn't stop it.

—Latrice, age twenty-seven

I got to the point that I couldn't come home. I would get totally paranoid. I would call my husband and tell him I

*didn't know what I was going to do. I had been put on a
lot of antidepressant medications and I was storing all kinds
of stuff. I got to the point one day that I was going to a
parking garage and I was going to kill myself. I wrote a
letter, I was storing pills in the glove compartment, I had
everything in there. But I couldn't find a place to park. It
happened to be a day when the place was crowded and I
couldn't get a private spot to park. And when things like
that happened, when I was getting to the end and my plan
was unraveling, I would really fall apart. The day I was
hospitalized, I was in my therapist's office and I just lost it.
He called my husband and said, "She's got to go into the
hospital." And I realized then I needed to go to the hospital,
too. I knew it was coming to that.*

—*Celeste, age forty*

These are the voices of major depression. The feelings these
women describe transcend sadness and the blues. These feelings of utter despair, hopelessness, and pain are the hallmarks
of major depression. Once ill, these women were robbed of
their ability to face the day. They were unable to do their work
or care for themselves and their families. They lost their zest
for life.

Major depression is by far the most severe of the depressive
disorders. It is diagnosed when a person has one or more depressive episodes—periods of distinct symptoms that indicate
depression—that last at least two weeks. A depressive episode
may gradually develop over a few days or weeks, or it may seem
to hit you out of the blue, as it did with Latrice. It may start
with a feeling of vague but persistent sadness or insidious apathy. Things that are normally engaging and fun seem blah;
nothing holds your interest anymore. Appetite and sleep patterns change. A sense of hopelessness may overtake you. It becomes physically difficult, if not impossible, to get out of bed.
As the depression worsens, the symptoms become over-

whelming. You think nothing will ever change, that you will always feel this way. You may start to think about suicide. You feel as if you have fallen into a deep pit, and you can't claw your way out of it. Depression can make even the strongest, most self-assured sister feel as if she can do nothing right and that there is no point in trying.

What Is a Depressive Episode?

The signs and symptoms of a depressive episode are distinct and fairly easy to recognize once you know what they are. Of course, not everyone experiences depression by the book. Some clinically depressed people have slightly different, less common symptoms. Mental health professionals look for at least five of the following symptoms when diagnosing a depressive episode:

Depressed or sad mood most of the day, nearly every day. Most depressed people report feeling extremely sad, and often they can't pinpoint any particular reason. As Latrice described it, "It just came out of nowhere." Others initially become sad as a result of some specific event, but the sadness mushrooms and gets out of control. Nona, thirty-one, became depressed after a boyfriend told her he was no longer in love with her. "I was heartbroken, but at first I thought, *You feel really horrible now, but that's to be expected. It'll get better.* And it didn't. I woke up crying every day. Some nights I'd cry for hours at a time—like from midnight till four in the morning. This went on for weeks. I knew this wasn't just about this man. This was something else."

Little or no interest in normal activities, even those that usually bring pleasure (anhedonia). People suffering from depression often feel as if they are walking around in a fog. They can't seem to get excited over anything, even things that would normally make them happy. Hobbies, exercise, hanging out with friends, even sex—nothing holds their interest. Elaine, sixty-nine, loves reading mysteries, and typically reads a book a week. When she is depressed, however, she can't read at all. "I don't even want to pick up a book," she says. "All I can do is sit and watch television, and I don't enjoy that, either."

Significant weight loss or weight gain without trying in a short span of time. Many depressed people find that they have no appetite, and that food has little taste. They eat next to nothing and may lose more than 5 percent of their body weight—say, dropping from 140 to near 130 pounds—in a month or less. Unfortunately, friends and family often fail to recognize this rapid weight loss as a problem, especially in women. They may be more likely to think the loss is attractive and compliment the woman on it than to think something is wrong.

Not all depressed people lose weight, however. A significant number eat *more* when they are depressed and put on weight very quickly. Food may become a comfort for them. The thing to watch out for is any sudden change in appetite or eating habits—either eating too much or too little. Either could be a sign of depression.

Inability to sleep (insomnia) or sleeping too much (hypersomnia)—almost every day. Sleep problems are another very common complaint of depressed people. Most, like Keisha, twenty-four, have *terminal insomnia*: they wake up after a few hours and can't fall asleep again. "I would go to sleep, but I would wake up two to three hours before I had to get up and I couldn't get back to sleep," Keisha recalls. Others find that they have a hard time falling asleep at night because they become overwhelmed by their feelings. Elaine remembers lying awake at night thinking about how awful she felt her life was. "At night, these horrible thoughts would start coming to me, over and over. They would tell me how everything had gone wrong, how I had messed everything up, how I should just end it all and kill myself. I couldn't turn my mind off." Since she couldn't get to sleep at night, Elaine would often sleep most of the day.

Slowed speech and/or movement (or agitated speech and/or movement). Depressed people often describe this feeling as being "weighted down" or "moving through quicksand." It can be physically difficult to move around as you normally would. It may take you longer to complete your thoughts and sentences, or you may speak more quietly than you usually do. Conversely, some depressed people become anxious and agitated. They may find it hard to sit still and may develop habits like hand-wringing, pacing, or constantly pulling their hair.

Fatigue or loss of energy. This is an almost universal symptom of depression. The majority of depressed people report feeling extremely tired most of the time, even when they do get enough sleep. Many continue to perform at work or school, though they usually let something else go—like their personal needs or physical appearance—because they simply don't have the energy to take care of everything they normally do. Even the smallest tasks seem to take superhuman effort. Renee remembers being unable to get out of bed for a week. When she did get up, she felt extremely tired, as if "someone was pressing me into the ground."

Feelings of worthlessness or excessive or inappropriate guilt. Depressed people usually believe that they are the cause of all their troubles. They blame themselves for things that they could not possibly control, and conclude that they are worthless and deserve anything bad that happens to them. They often feel responsible and guilty for other people's problems, as well. When Elaine was depressed, she not only blamed herself for her past relationship problems and current financial woes, she felt as if she were somehow responsible for all of the problems in her two daughters' lives, too.

Inability to think, concentrate, or make decisions. Depressed people often complain that they can't keep their minds on things they need to do. As a college student, Nona found it impossible to study when she became depressed. "I sat and stared at the words on the pages, but I couldn't make any sense of it," she says. Memory problems are also a common complaint.

Recurrent thoughts of death or suicide, making a plan to commit suicide, and previous suicide attempts. These are clear indicators that a person is seriously depressed. Anyone who talks about suicide or says things like "You'd be better off if I weren't around" should be taken seriously. If you feel suicidal, get to an emergency room immediately.

If a person has been in a sad or depressed mood or has lost interest or pleasure in her regular activities; has had at least four or more of the above symptoms for two weeks or more; and the symptoms have made it difficult or impossible for her to work, go to school, take care of herself or her family, or otherwise live her life, her doctor or therapist will likely diagnose depression.

Although the symptoms must last at least two weeks in order to be classified as a depressive episode, an untreated episode usually lasts about six months. Most depressive episodes will self-limit—that is, end on their own, without treatment. With treatment, however, most of these episodes could end a lot sooner. Also, without treatment, subsequent episodes are likely to be more severe. In a significant minority of cases, perhaps 20 to 30 percent, some depressive symptoms will remain for several months to years. These cases are said to be in *partial remission*. Severe depressive episodes are more likely to go into partial remission than to end completely. About 5 to 10 percent of all depressed people continue to experience all their depressive symptoms for two years or more, and are considered *chronically depressed*. Anyone who has two or more depressive episodes is said to have *recurrent* depression.

Major depression can strike at any age, although the average age for a first depressive episode is about twenty-five. (Often, people experience some depressive symptoms much earlier, but the full-blown illness does not emerge until early adulthood.) Some people have just one depressive episode and never experience another. Most, however, have recurrent episodes, sometimes separated by many years, sometimes in clusters, and sometimes increasing in frequency with age. The more depressive episodes a person has had, the more likely it is that she will have another. Fifty to 60 percent of people who have had one depressive episode will have a second, 70 percent of those who have had a second will have a third, and 90 percent of those who have a third depressive episode will have a fourth. About 5 to 10 percent of people who have a depressive episode will go on to develop a bipolar disorder, discussed later in this chapter.

Dysthymic Disorder

Dysthymic disorder (also called *dysthymia*) is a chronic depressive disorder that affects 3 to 5 percent of the adult population. As with major depression, most dysthymia sufferers are women. Dysthymia is also more common among young and unmarried people and among people with low incomes. People with dysthymia experience some of the symptoms of major depression, but they usually aren't as intense. More important, however, is the fact that dysthymic disorder is not episodic like major depressive disorder. With dysthymic disorder, the symptoms are ever-present, so much so that they come to be thought of as part of the sufferer's personality.

Dysthymic disorder is diagnosed when a person is in a depressed mood for most of the day, more days than not, for two years or more, and has at least two of the following symptoms:

- Poor appetite or overeating
- Insomnia or sleeping too much
- Low energy or fatigue
- Low self-esteem

- Poor concentration or difficulty making decisions
- Feelings of hopelessness

People suffering from dysthymia are often thought of as pessimistic, negative, self-critical, and unmotivated. They are chronically unhappy, lethargic, and dissatisfied. Because their symptoms last for so long and are such a part of their day-to-day reality, people with dysthymia are more likely to be written off by others as having a bad attitude or a negative view of life. People with dysthymia tend to believe that their chronic bleak outlook is a part of their personality and explain it by saying, "This is just how I am." They often have very low self-esteem because they blame themselves for their inability to get motivated, be sociable, or enjoy life. Few are likely to recognize their complaints as symptomatic of a treatable mental disorder.

Dysthymia sufferers rarely talk about or attempt suicide. The long-term nature of their illness often interferes with their personal relationships and job performance, however. People with dysthymia are less likely to get married, more likely to get divorced, and are often unemployed or underemployed. They are caught in a self-perpetuating cycle: their illness makes them negative and withdrawn, so they find it hard to establish and maintain relationships. This confirms what they already believe—that they are hopeless and worthless, and that nothing will ever get better. The depressed mood—and the cycle—continue. The chronic nature of dysthymia often leads those with the disorder to try to mask their pain with alcohol and other drugs, as well.

Dysthymia usually starts early in life, often in childhood or during the teenage years. People who develop dysthymia before they are twenty-one years old often develop major depression. In general, about 10 percent of people with dysthymia will develop major depression in any given year. People suffering from both major depression and dysthymia are said to have *double depression,* a condition that is difficult to treat.

Other Depressive Disorders

A person who has a few depressive symptoms, but not enough to be diagnosed with major depressive disorder or dysthymic disorder, might be suffering from one of the other, lesser-known depressions. These include minor depressive disorder, recurrent brief depressive disorder, the controversial premenstrual dysphoric disorder, and postpartum depression. Though these disorders are not yet official DSM-IV diagnoses, they may become so with the next revision of the DSM. They do seem to be distinct disorders.

Minor and Recurrent Brief Depressions

Minor depression differs from major depression in severity: it lasts just as long as major depression (at least two weeks), but the symptoms are fewer and less extreme, and the person with minor depression is more able to function. While major depression renders most people incapable of getting through their normal routines, minor depression makes those routines more difficult, but not impossible. As with both major depression and dysthymia, the primary symptom of minor depression is depressed mood. At least two but fewer than five of the other symptoms of depression must be present as well (loss of interest or pleasure; significant weight loss or gain; sleep problems, psychomotor agitation or retardation, fatigue, inability to think or concentrate, feelings of worthlessness or hopelessness, and thoughts of death or suicide).

Minor depression may be as common as major depression, but the research on this disorder is limited, and no one knows for sure. It is also thought to occur more commonly in women than men. Distinguishing between a mild case of major depression and minor depression can be hard—and some would say pointless. There is nothing to suggest that the treatment for minor depression should be any different than that for major depression, and for that reason the distinction is somewhat academic.

Recurrent brief depressions are like major depressions in every way except duration. The number and severity of the symptoms is the same, but recurrent brief depressions last less than two weeks (usually from two to four days). These brief depressive episodes must recur at least once a month for a year in order to be diagnosed as recurrent brief depressions. Unlike minor depressions, these brief depressions are debilitating, and they do interfere with the ability to function. A person with recurrent brief depressions may not be able to work at all on the days she is depressed. The recurrences can't be associated with a woman's menstrual cycle, however. If they are, she is diagnosed with premenstrual dysphoric disorder.

To date, there has been little research on this depressive disorder. It seems to affect people of all ages, though it is thought to be more common among young adults. Estimates are that about 5 percent of the population suffers from recurrent brief depression, but close to 10 percent of people in their twenties do.

Premenstrual Dysphoric Disorder

Premenstrual dysphoric disorder (PMDD) is perhaps the most controversial of the depressive disorders. Not everyone agrees that it is an actual mental disorder. Some researchers (especially women researchers) worry that it will be used as an excuse to discriminate against women and that it gives credence to the old myth that women are hostages to their hormones. Others argue that some women do experience a distinct set of depressive symptoms during the luteal phase of their menstrual cycles (the time between ovulation and the onset of the menstrual period), and that this should be diagnosed as a depressive disorder. Sarah Gehlert, Ph.D., a social work researcher at the University of Chicago's School of Social Service Administration, is conducting a national study of thousands of women to help determine whether or not PMDD is a true psychiatric disorder.

The symptoms of premenstrual dysphoric disorder are slightly different from those of the other depressive disorders. In fact, they are what most of us know as premenstrual syndrome (PMS). In order to be considered PMDD, symptoms must be severe enough to interfere with your daily functioning and relationships. The symptoms of PMDD, which appear one to two weeks before your period, are:

- Depressed mood, feelings of hopelessness, or self-deprecating thoughts (put-downs)
- Anxiety, tension, or feeling on edge
- Extreme sensitivity (for instance, crying easily and without much provocation)
- Anger, irritability, or increased conflicts in personal relationships
- Loss of interest in usual activities
- Tiredness or lack of energy
- Change in appetite, overeating, or specific food cravings
- Sleep problems (sleeping too much or insomnia)
- Feeling overwhelmed or out of control
- Physical symptoms such as breast tenderness or swelling, bloating, headaches, or joint or muscle pain

So, what's the difference between premenstrual dysphoric disorder and plain old PMS? Good question. How many women have PMDD? How should PMDD be treated? These are also good questions. One study found that about 40 percent of women have mild symptoms (what we would probably call PMS), but only 2 to 3 percent have symptoms severe enough to truly disrupt their lives. Severe PMDD seems to be treatable about 65 percent of the time, and certain antidepressant drugs seem to be most effective. PMDD usually starts when a woman is in her late twenties, and it probably gets worse with age. As many as 30 percent of women with PMDD have also had a major depressive episode at some point in their lives, and women with PMDD are at higher risk of having future major depressive episodes.

Seasonal Affective Disorder

People who tend to become depressed at a specific time of year are said to have a seasonal pattern to their depression. Depressions that begin in winter and end in spring are known by the popular term *seasonal affective disorder* (SAD). Though seasonal depressions can occur at the start of any season, the fall/winter onset ones are more common. DSM-IV does not use the term seasonal affective disorder. Instead, seasonal depressions are classified as a specific type of major depressive disorder. This may change with more research, however. Some studies suggest that seasonal depressions may be quite different from other types of depression (for one thing, they can be treated very successfully with light therapy—exposure to full-spectrum light—while other forms of depression do not respond to light therapy). As with all other depressive disorders, seasonal depressions are more common in women than in men.

Postpartum Depression

It is a well-known fact that most women experience a letdown after having a baby. After all the anticipation and excitement of pregnancy (and the hard work of labor and delivery), a few days of these baby blues is to be expected. Between 50 and 80 percent of women have the baby blues after giving birth.

For 10 to 20 percent of new mothers, the postpartum period brings a more serious problem: depression. These depressions can be either major or minor depressive episodes. Women who have had depressive episodes before pregnancy are more likely to have postpartum depression, and women who suffer from postpartum depression are likely to have future depressive episodes. Who is at risk for postpartum depression? While there is probably a biological underpinning to the illness, women who have significant life stresses like money problems are more at risk. So are women who have serious marital or relationship problems, or who have had complicated pregnancies, miscarriages, or stillbirths. Some psychologists suggest that many women with postpartum depression may have unresolved feelings about being a mother—perhaps they didn't want to become pregnant or they may feel trapped in an unhappy marriage by motherhood.

Whatever the cause, postpartum depression is extremely distressing to the new mother (who may feel guilt and shame because she is not more excited about the baby), and her partner, family, and friends (who may tell her the depression is all in her head and feel she is being self-indulgent). Further complicating matters is the fact that many ob-gyns and psychiatrists fail to recognize postpartum depression because they, too, confuse it with the baby blues. These well-meaning but misled doctors may tell the depressed mother that the problem is indeed in her head, thus failing to treat what may be a serious depression with long-term consequences for the mother, the child, and the parents' relationship.

Women with postpartum depression have true depressive symptoms that begin within a few days to a few weeks after giving birth. Symptoms include:

- Depressed mood
- Obsessive worrying about the baby
- Panic attacks
- Disturbed sleep (other than that caused by the baby's schedule)
- Poor energy
- Poor concentration
- Feelings of guilt and inadequacy

Postpartum depression is obviously upsetting and dangerous to the mother, but it can also affect the baby. Maternal withdrawal and overprotectiveness common to postpartum depression can interfere with mother-infant bonding and can cause anger, withdrawal, reduced activity, and developmental problems in the baby. Postpartum depression is also associated with behavior problems later in childhood. For these reasons, as well as for the health and safety of the mother, postpartum depression must be diagnosed and treated early.

A small number of women (perhaps 1 out of every 1,000 postpartum women) develop *postpartum psychosis,* a more serious psychiatric disorder that can lead a mother to commit suicide or even kill her baby. Postpartum psychosis is not a mood disorder, but it is mentioned here because it can be confused with postpartum depression. New mothers who become increasingly agitated, have wildly fluctuating moods, disturbed sleep, periods of confusion, and who seem paranoid, have delusions or hallucinations, or hear voices, may have postpartum psychosis. Postpartum psychosis is considered a psychiatric emergency, and women with these symptoms should be closely supervised by a psychiatrist. Hospitalization is often necessary to prevent suicide attempts or attempts to harm the baby.

The Bipolar Disorders: Bipolar I and II and Cyclothymia

While they are also classified as mood disorders, bipolar disorders differ from unipolar disorders in one basic way: people with bipolar disorders experience mania. Mania is a period of intense and uncharacteristic activity and euphoria. When in a manic phase, sufferers are on an irrepressible high. Some say they feel as if they are flying. A person is considered to be in a manic episode if she experiences an uncharacteristic feeling of euphoria or elevated mood (or feels unusually irritable and angry) for at least two weeks, and has at least five of these symptoms:

- A feeling of self-importance or inflated self-esteem
- A decreased need for sleep (feeling rested after having just a few hours of sleep a night when you normally need eight)
- Talking rapidly, becoming extremely talkative, and monopolizing conversations
- Feeling as if the mind is racing—that thoughts come too quickly to keep up with them
- Increased activity at work or school
- Increased sex drive
- Feeling restless or unable to keep still
- Impulsive behavior, like becoming promiscuous, going on buying sprees, or making rash business decisions

Though people with bipolar disorder sometimes get a lot accomplished during a manic phase, these periods can be tremendously destructive. People suffering from mania may damage their relationships by picking up strangers and sleeping around. They may spend themselves into bankruptcy or use drugs excessively. Those with severe mania are more likely to commit spouse abuse, child abuse, or become violent in other ways. Mania, like depression, sends a person spinning out of control, but instead of spiraling into self-loathing and depression, the person with mania soars into self-aggrandizement, hyperactivity, or uncontrolled rage.

Most of the time, the mania is only half of the story. Sixty percent of people with bipolar I disorder eventually crash into the depressive phase of their illness. In most cases—about 60 to 70 percent of the time—manic episodes occur immediately before or after depressive episodes. Also, once you've had one manic episode, you are almost certain to have another—90 percent of people who have a single manic episode have subsequent ones. And 15 percent of people with bipolar disorder, like those with unipolar depression, end up committing suicide. The pain of being two different people—one withdrawn and depressed, one larger than life and out of control, and neither one the true self—is often too much to take.

Some people with bipolar disorder have less dramatic manic phases, called *hypomania*, along with major depressive episodes. These people are said to have *bipolar II disorder*. Hypomanic episodes are shorter than manic episodes, and have fewer manic symptoms to a lesser degree. People who have many periods of hypomania and mild to moderate depressive symptoms are said to have *cyclothymia*. Cyclothymia, like dysthymia, is a chronic disorder, and symptoms must be present for two years or more in order for cyclothymia to be diagnosed. This disorder usually begins in adolescence or early adulthood, and is equally common in men and women. People with cyclothymia have a 15 to 50 percent chance of developing a more serious bipolar disorder.

What Depression Isn't

The Blues

Black women *know* the blues, and know them well. Blues mamas like Bessie Smith and Ma Rainey sang 'em and lived 'em. From the beginning, the blues were more than just music for Black people: they were testimony, support, and salve. Blues was born in the unforgiving rural South, to people whose physical, emotional, and psychic pain received little or no attention. Blues was Black folks' doctor. As poet O. P. Adisa writes, "Blues is medicine because it is not meant to depress or pull one down—it has the opposite effect. The blues heals." But while the blues is a major part of (and expression of) the Black experience, depression is not.

Though blues singers like Ma Rainey and Bessie Smith sang

blues about everything from sex to sorrow, many Black women identify with their so-called independent women's blues—songs that depicted Black women picking up the pieces after something had gone wrong and moving on with their lives. From these mothers of the blues we learn that blues aren't necessarily a bad thing. Black women use the blues as a way of processing, a kind of self-therapy that allows us to state and affirm that, yes, life has dealt us a raw deal, but it's a temporary thing. It will resolve itself.

The blues starts out with bad news—a love has left, money is short, times are hard—then proposes solutions. By the end, there's new hope, there are new possibilities. Bessie Smith's "Young Woman Blues" is a perfect example of the problem-solving, healing function of the blues:

> *Woke up this mornin', when chickens was crowing for day*
> *Felt on the right side of my pillow, my man had gone away*
> *On his pillow he left a note, reading I'm sorry, you got*
>   *my goat*
> *No time to marry, no time to settle down*

This woman clearly woke up to some bad news. But she got to thinking . . .

> *I'm a young woman, and ain't done runnin' 'round*
> *I'm a young woman, and ain't done runnin' 'round*
> *Some people call me a hobo, some call me a bum*
> *Nobody knows my name, nobody knows what I've done*
> *I'm as good as any woman in your town*

By the end of the song, she has worked it out:

> *See that long, lonesome road, Lord knows it's gotta end*
> *and I'm a good woman, and I can get plenty men*

Evelyn Barbee, a researcher at the Boston College School of Nursing, found that Black women see the blues as a healing time, a time of transition and a signal to take some time out for themselves. Barbee recognizes that the blues—the music and the state of mind—are informed by Black culture. While some might view having the blues as a sign of mental distress, Barbee says Black women see the blues as a time to go inside themselves for a bit of self-healing.

According to the women in Barbee's study, the blues are a point on the continuum between just feeling down and true depression. The blues come along when your mind is troubled and you just can't shake it, when things just aren't going as planned. A great many things can bring on the blues: problems with relationships or work, worries about children or money, adjusting to being single or getting married, even just thinking about the Black woman's lot in life. The blues overcome you like stormy weather, and while they don't drown you, they sure do make everything look gray for a while.

The blues may look like a more serious depression while you're in them. You're sad and apathetic. You feel tired, run-down, and may not want to get out of bed. You won't eat much, or you do nothing but eat. You're short-tempered and out of sorts. The things that usually make you happy simply aren't doing it for you now, and all you want to do is be by yourself. The difference between these depressive feelings and depression the illness is one of degree and duration. While having the blues feels bad, it is not an unbearable bad, and you know you'll emerge from them soon. With the blues, you still have perspective. With depression, perspective is skewed. The main difference between the blues and depression is hope.

While in the midst of the blues, a woman is forced to take an honest look at a problem that she may have been avoiding. You can believe that the woman in "Young Woman Blues" had problems with her man before that morning she woke up and found him gone. If she was like many Black women, she told herself she didn't have time to think about what might be wrong, what with her job and her children and her mother and who knows what else working her nerves. But his leaving stopped her in her tracks and made her face the fact that the relationship was no longer. No, it didn't feel good. But it was a necessary time of introspection. So she went into the blues, and while there, realized that she was a good woman who could find herself another man, if that was what she wanted. For this Black woman, as for many others, the blues was a regenerative, transformative experience.

Grief

Like the blues, grief is more than sadness. It is deeper, it is harder, and it can be infinitely more painful. It can take months, even a year or more, to truly move beyond grief. Still, it is not clinical depression.

Losing someone close, whether it is a parent, a sibling, a child, a friend, or a mate, is devastating. The death of a loved one can make you feel so out of control, so deeply sad, that you might wonder if you can—or want to—go on living. But, as with the blues, the difference between grief and depression is largely one of hope.

The day-to-day working through grief is exhausting, but, in a normal grief reaction, you get to a point where you know you will come through on the other side. There are five accepted stages of grief: denial and isolation, anger, bargaining, depression, and acceptance, although they aren't always experienced in that order. Most people experience each of these stages, but some may not.

When you first get the news that someone close to you has died, you may not want to believe it. We have all seen people, who, when they are told of a loved one's death, want to talk to the dead person, or who, weeks later, still speak of the deceased as if they are living. This denial is a type of shock reaction.

It is a form of self-protection that persists until people are emotionally ready to begin the work of grieving.

Once the mourning begins, anger sets in. You're angry with the person who died for leaving you. You wonder if the death is somehow your fault, if you did enough. You may be angry with doctors for not doing enough to keep your loved one alive. If the death was violent, you are certainly angry with the person who took your loved one's life (and if that person took his or her own life, the anger may be even more intense and difficult). You may even be angry with God. You may start to bargain: if you go to church every Sunday, maybe the person who died will come back to you, or no one else will die.

Soon, anger turns to sadness. Anger takes a lot of energy, and you can only keep it going for so long. Now you want to give up. You don't want to get out of bed. You cry all day, won't eat, can't sleep. Nothing—not even your favorite things—makes you feel better. You feel lost without the person who died. You aren't sure if you want to live without them, or if you can. This grief-related depression is normal, and usually isn't very severe and doesn't last very long. Yes, it feels horrible, but again, even with grief-related depression, there is hope. Eventually, you accept the death. You never forget, but you move on. You learn to deal with the loneliness, you let yourself be sad when you need to, and you get back to the business of living your life. This normal grief is necessary and temporary. Depression is something quite different.

ARE YOU DEPRESSED?

Are you wondering if you or someone close to you might be depressed? Do you agree with any of these statements?

1. I feel extremely sad, down in the dumps, or numb.
2. I don't enjoy the things that I used to.
3. I am losing weight even though I'm not on a diet (OR Eating is the only thing that seems to make me feel better).

4. I have trouble falling asleep or sleeping through the night (OR I am sleeping far more than I usually do).
5. I feel slowed down. My limbs feel heavy, like I'm under water.
6. I am restless and I can't keep still.
7. My mind isn't as clear as it used to be. I have trouble thinking, concentrating, and/or making decisions.
8. I feel tired all the time.
9. I am a worthless human being.
10. I deserve anything bad that happens to me.
11. I feel hopeless about the future.
12. Everyone would be better off if I weren't around.

If you agree with at least five of these statements (including numbers one and two), and you have been feeling this way for at least two weeks, you may be depressed. Talk to your primary care doctor and ask for a referral, or consult a mental health practitioner directly. (If you agree with statements 11 and 12, it is very important that you alert someone immediately.)

One reason Black women don't get treated for depression is that we often expect to feel sad, tired, and unable to think straight. How many Black women have sung "Nobody knows the trouble I've seen . . ." or "Soon will be done with the troubles of the world . . ." or "Sometimes I feel like a motherless child . . ."? Struggle and pain have often characterized Black women's lives more than love and joy. You may have looked at these questions and thought, *Yeah, and what else is new? All the Black women I know feel this way.* While all of us do feel sad, run-down, restless, or confused from time to time, no one should feel this way for too long. If you do, you are probably depressed. **Remember, Black women do not have to be depressed. It is not our lot in life.**

PART II

· · · · · · · · · ·

STRESS
AND DEPRESSION
IN BLACK WOMEN

2

• • • • • • •

The Mule of the World and Other Myths: How Stereotypes of Black Women Contribute to Depression

Sapphire. Mammy. Tragic mulatto wench. Workhorse, can swing an ax, lift a load, pick cotton with any man. A wonderful housekeeper. Excellent with children. Very clean. Very religious. A terrific mother. A great little singer and dancer and a devoted teacher and social worker. She's always had more opportunities than the Black man because she was no threat to the white man so he made it easy for her. But curiously enough, she frequently ends up on welfare. Nevertheless, she is more educated and makes more money than the Black man. She is more likely to be employed and more likely to be a professional than the Black man. And subsequently she provides the main support for the family. Not beautiful, rather hard looking unless she has some white blood, but then very beautiful. The Black ones are exotic though, great in bed, tigers. And very fertile. If she is middle class she tends to be uptight about sex, prudish. She is hard on and unsupportive of Black men, domineering, castrating. She tends to wear the pants around the house. Very strong. Sorrow rolls off her brow like so much rain. Tough, unfeminine, opposed to women's rights movements, considers herself already liberated. Nevertheless, unworldly. Definitely not a dreamer, rigid, inflexible, uncompassionate, lacking any

*goals more imaginative than a bucket of fried chicken and
a good fuck.*

—Michele Wallace, *Black Macho
and the Myth of the Superwoman* (Verso, 1990)

Who is this woman Michele Wallace describes? Is she anyone
you know? Is she you? Like it or not, the Black woman of Wallace's pen is the Black woman many people think you are or
want you to be. Even worse, that Black woman is the person
many of us have internalized and believe we are or should be.
How many times have you been told who you are by other
people? How many times have your ideas been questioned,
your desires ridiculed, your abilities doubted because you are
a Black woman? How many times do we limit ourselves because
we have been taught that something we do, say, or want is out
of our reach, not for us or about us, or something we shouldn't
want if we're to be good Black women?

Every day, Black women wake up and face a world bent on
defining them in constraining and demeaning ways. We turn
on the television news and see ourselves as drug-addicted welfare mothers of innumerable neglected children, and as either
stoic or hysterical mourners at the funerals of our brothers,
sisters, lovers, and children. We listen to music that often portrays us as accessories, good only for sex (albeit good sex), who,
once we've overstayed our welcome, become bitching drains
on the wallet, distractions from the real business of life. We go
to work, where we are seen as the exception (intelligent and
hardworking) to the rule (dumb and lazy) when we know we
are the rule; or where we're commonly known as the affirmative
action experiment, always expected to prove ourselves the inferior talent everyone suspects we are. Even family and friends
tell us who we are and can hope to be, sometimes causing
doubt and wariness when they only meant to protect us from
the inevitable hurts incurred by being a Black woman.

How do we learn who we are and what's expected of us?

Who teaches us the lessons of life as a Black woman? And what do these lessons tell us about what we can and should expect for ourselves?

Call Me What You Like: Old and New Stereotypes of Black Women

Try as it might, American popular culture has never been able to rid itself of the problem of the Black woman. Since we first landed here in 1619, the effort to define us has been unfailing. Too "other" to be true woman (too dark, too strong, too different), we have been cast as both hopelessly ineffectual and dangerously strong, hilarious and threatening, desirable and despicable. Who and what does the popular culture say we are? Any number of things, but rarely truly human.

Mammy

The mammy is one of the oldest and most enduring stereotypes of Black women. She is ubiquitous—found on everything from your pancake mix (though now with a new '90s 'do) to the local news. Her popularity is perhaps explained by the fact that the mammy is a throwback to a time when everyone knew his or her place, when public discourse was unmarred by such things as protest and calls for civil rights. The Black woman's place during this time was as mammy, wet nurse, and caretaker to white America.

The mammy stereotype is rooted in the history of slavery, when an actual mammy was central to the efficient management of the master's household. She fed, coddled, and disciplined the master's children (often actually nursing them along with her own), ran his kitchen, and was maidservant to his wife. Since she was so often present in the master's home, the woman chosen as mammy had to be the least sexually appealing so as to appease the mistress, and was therefore usually obese, dark-skinned, and broad-featured—in short, the antithesis of the American idea of beauty and womanhood. Mammy was often the loyal confidant of the mistress, whom she served dutifully. Although she was trusted with child rearing and household tasks, she was certainly not seen as fully human. She was amusing to those she served, and sometimes had to be put in her place. Most of all, Mammy was compliant. She trusted that the master and mistress would take care of her if she just did her job well, and she strongly defended them against other slaves who were subject to harsher treatment. She was loyal to the death.

Today we most often see the mammy stereotype on television, in sitcoms like the '80s *Gimme a Break*, or in advertisements for pancake mix and household cleaners. On the surface, these women happily take care of other people's children and clean their homes. They solve the other adults' problems, unravel their messes, and help them make sense of their complicated lives. But they rarely take care of themselves. The new mammies almost never have social lives or friends of their own, and they never have successful romantic relationships. The message is that they are happy only when serving others— particularly whites. Loving, balanced, equal adult relationships are not for Mammy, so if she knows what's best, she won't even wish for them.

The mammy stereotype is indelibly imprinted on the American psyche, so much so that we expect some aspects of mammylike behavior from all Black women, whether they fit the physical description of Mammy or not. Our popular definition of the good Black woman most often begins with service to someone other than the self: a good sister is a devoted wife, a selfless and giving mother, the one who holds the family and community together. While this description of the good sister is certainly flattering in some ways and rings true to our experience, it does not acknowledge the basic fact that the Black woman also has to be good to herself, that her needs are at least as important as those of her partner, children, and community. Popular culture still expects us to be the uncomplaining, congenial, deferential problem solver, the traditional mammy stereotype without the head rag.

Elaine tells of coworkers who expected mammy behavior of her, and let her know they were disappointed when she didn't deliver. "I received a less-than-positive review from my supervisor, which I didn't understand. I knew I had done my job well. When I went in to question the review, my supervisor, a white woman, told me that several of my coworkers complained that I was intimidating and hard to get along with. I knew what she meant—I didn't make them feel good, I didn't make them laugh, put them at ease, socialize with them at lunch. I was there to do a job, but I was being rated on how comfortable I made the whites I worked with feel."

In short, Elaine's coworkers didn't quite know what to do with a Black woman whose main concern was not how *they* felt. Women, no matter what race, are often expected to be deferential on the job, and those who aren't or who openly display ambition or assertiveness are quickly labeled bitchy or cold. But Black women who fail to placate their coworkers are often labeled this way by both white men and women, because Americans have been conditioned, through centuries of stereotyping, to expect the Black woman to be the shoulder for all to lean and cry on, the one who makes everything all right.

The Mammy stereotype tells others:

- Black women are here to serve and nurture you.
- Black women are good at solving other people's problems, though they're not so great at solving their own.
- Black women get all their fulfillment in life from helping others.

The mammy stereotype tells Black women:

- We are responsible for everyone else's well-being.
- We don't need and shouldn't expect nurturing.
- Our own needs are secondary to others' needs.
- We should feel guilty when we put our own needs before those of others.

Sapphire

> *My aunt Alma was always following my uncle around, nagging him to death. He would totally ignore her until he just couldn't take it anymore, and then he'd turn to her and say, "Hush up, woman." We all laughed when he did that. Now I can't believe how easily he—and the rest of us—dismissed everything she had to say. I'm sure she nagged so much because she thought it was the only way to get him to listen.*
>
> *—Nona*

According to the prevailing stereotypes, when Black women aren't serving, we're complaining. Sapphire—actually the name of a loquacious and perennially dissatisfied Black female character on the *Amos & Andy* television show of the 1950s—is the archetypal nagging Black woman. Sapphire was famous for her unceasing verbal combat with her television husband, Kingfish. She pointed out his every flaw and generally cut him down for being, in her opinion, lazy, no-count, good-for-nothing, trifling, and overall a sorry excuse for a man. Sapphire punctuated this litany with a fast-moving neck and an ever-wagging finger. Carping, emasculating, and shrill, Sapphire was never taken seriously. The most attention she got for her trouble was an acknowledgment that she was "always running her mouth."

In the '90s we laugh at our own versions of Sapphire, from Harriet, the quick-with-a-quip mother on *Family Matters*, to Martin Lawrence's Shanaynay, the woman he loves to hate on his eponymous television show, to any number of young, tough, female pop artists featured in music videos. But are these images really funny? They show us a Black woman who is at best dissatisfied and desperately trying to gain some control, and at worst bitter and hateful. The Sapphire stereotype says that Black women can never be satisfied, and the subtext is that one shouldn't even try. Perhaps most damaging, Sapphire's constant tongue-lashing tells us that this is the way Black women communicate—by cutting down and playing the dozens. How many of us grew up with mothers who told us—and our fathers—"Black men ain't worth ———"? How many of us were castigated with lines like "Get your lazy Black butt over here?" Often stripped of respect by their interactions with the world, our mothers sometimes learned to demand it through Sapphire-style verbal put-downs. The Sapphire stereotype is ill equipped for tender conversation, for secret sharing, for loving advice. She is the woman who would tell you "it's your own damn fault" if you lost your job or got hit by your husband. While some may see Sapphire's acrid verbal style as a cover-up for her own insecurities (and often when women behave this way, that is the case), the Sapphire stereotype of Black women denies sisters' warmth and humanity, and when this style of communication is adopted, it prevents us from forming warm bonds with those we care about. The Sapphire stereotype tells us that we need to be verbally aggressive and combative if we want to be heard at all.

The Sapphire stereotype tells others:

- Black women are loud, obnoxious, and nagging, and it is OK to ignore them.
- Black women are emasculating, and they need to be put in their proper place.

- Black women are never satisfied with anything you do. They aren't worth trying to satisfy.
- Black women never listen.

The Sapphire stereotype tells Black women:

- No one will pay attention to us unless we make them.
- We are easy to ignore.
- Ignoring us is funny.
- What we think or say has little value.
- In order to be listened to, we must make ourselves heard any way we can.
- Loving, gentle communication doesn't get us anywhere.

Tragic Mulatto

The tragic mulatto stereotype was, in its heyday, the answer to the question: "What about the children?" She, like her namesake the mule, was a horrible trick played on nature. The tragic mulatto grew out of a time when it was impossible to imagine that anything good could come out of a sexual relationship (it was never love) between a Black person and a white person. The tragic mulatto, historically, was the product of the rape of a Black woman by a white man, either her slave master or the head of the household in which she worked as a domestic. Her life was doomed from the start. Light-skinned with flowing, silken hair, she often passed for white. But she was never truly happy, of course, because she wasn't truly white. And therein lies the tragedy. The tragic mulatto was tainted.

If she chose not to pass, the Black community could make life difficult for the tragic mulatto, too. Judged a temptress, other Black women didn't trust her. They called her snotty, hincty, uppity, saditty; they said, "She thinks she's cute." Never fitting in anywhere, the tragic mulatto drank herself into oblivion, threw herself out of windows, or disappeared, like the protagonists in Nella Larsen's novels *Quicksand* and *Passing*, and Fredi Washington in *Imitation of Life*.

Today, this stereotype most often manifests itself as negative views of light-skinned Black women, who may or may not be what we now call biracial. When we see light-skinned Black women in movies or on television (which isn't often) they are likely to be airheaded and confused, class-conscious and materialistic, or manipulative (or manipulated) sex objects. (Think of bubble-headed Hillary on *The Fresh Prince of Bel Air* and BAP [Black American Princess]-extraordinaire Whitley on *A Different World.*) Rarely do we see a together, light-skinned sister in the media. And even when we do, we are likely to ask her to prove her Blackness, because, according to the stereotype, if she's light, she'd rather be white. Sisters all over the country threw up their hands when Vanessa Williams was crowned Miss America, complaining, "Why couldn't they get a *real* Black woman?" What was the dethroning of the fair-skinned, hazel-eyed Williams if not a version of the tragic mulatto story?

The strength of the tragic mulatto stereotype and the color- and class-consciousness it fostered are testaments to the efficacy of both segregation and the divide-and-conquer strategy. The tragic mulatto stereotype was invented to keep Blacks and whites from intermarrying and having children. But the children were born, and often were afforded privileges by whites that other Black folk were not. They were told by white society that they were better than other Blacks but not as good as whites. They were often well-educated and assumed positions of power within the Black community. They quickly learned the value of light skin from whites, and they often socialized among themselves and married each other to perpetuate their light skin. The divisions between biracial, light-skinned, and dark-skinned Blacks is a historical fact. The tragic mulatto, the woman who is too confused to be happy, is not. What's tragic is that we still use this stereotype to define—and divide—ourselves and each other.

The tragic mulatto stereotype tells others:

- Children of interracial unions will never be happy.
- Light-skinned Black women are exotic, emotional, and passionate.
- Light-skinned women want to be white.
- Nothing good can ever come of mixing the races.

The tragic mulatto stereotype tells Black women:

- Light-skinned Black women are not to be trusted.
- Light-skinned Black women are prettier and more desirable than darker-skinned women.
- Light-skinned women have to prove themselves Black enough.
- Nothing good can ever come of mixing with whites.
- There is only one right way to be Black.

Jezebel/Bad Black Woman

Jezebel, a brown-skinned combination of Sapphire and the tragic mulatto, is all about sex. She's stacked and knows how to use what she's got. She works her sexuality like a voodoo charm—if she wants a man, he's powerless against her. Jezebel is the hypersexed Black woman of slave masters' imaginations and good church-goin' sisters' nightmares. She has men in the palm of her hand and anywhere else she wants them. What's more, Jezebel is alive and well in the popular media. She is the gold-digging hot young thing eager to sleep with the drug kingpin played by Wesley Snipes in the movie *New Jack City*; she's TV's purring Sandra Clark (played by Jackeé) on *227*; she's the "ho" in many rap songs.

The Jezebel stereotype reduces Black women to the equivalent of dogs in heat. This stereotype says we are animalistic in our desire, unable to control our sex drives or the effect they have on men. We are dangerous to white and Black men alike, for they all fall into our trap. The Jezebel stereotype warps the sensuous nature of Black women, often making it difficult for us to express our sexuality in healthy ways. Instead of celebrating our sexual selves, the prevalence of the Jezebel stereotype can make us either want to hide this part of us, since acknowledgment of our sexuality is akin to admitting to the stereotype, or use it as a weapon to keep men or get attention we might not otherwise get, attention we often mistake for or try to substitute for love.

The Jezebel stereotype tells others:

- Black women are all about sex.
- Black women use sex to get what they want.
- Men are powerless against the sexual wiles of the Black woman (so if you rape, beat, or sexually humiliate her, it's not your fault).

The Jezebel stereotype tells Black women:

- People always see us as sexual objects.
- Sex can get you what you want.
- Other Black women are not to be trusted (they are always out to get your man).
- Men are powerless against the sexual wiles of the Black woman (so if we are raped, beaten, or sexually humiliated, we brought it on ourselves).
- It is safest to keep your sexuality under wraps.

The Bitter Sister
The bitter sister didn't have a name until 1992. She became embodied, for many who watched the news that year, in the

person of Anita Hill. The bitter sister is a contemporary take on the Sapphire stereotype, one that has flourished as Black women attain more professional positions in society and otherwise "overstep their bounds." According to this stereotype, the bitter sister is bitter because she dared to think she could follow the white world's rules and they would work for her. She went to school, got a degree (or degrees), worked in a law firm or bank or school, and got to thinking she was all that. In other words, she forgot her place. And when things didn't go her way, she got bitter and lashed out at the only person she could—the Black man. Consequently, the bitter sister wants to tear the Black man down and will go to all lengths to do it.

A troubling number of Blacks, men and women alike, bought this picture of Anita Hill as the spurned, uptight law professor on a mission to destroy a brother. Portraying Black working and professional women in this manner demeans the very real concerns and problems they must grapple with. Black professional women face the same institutional racism Black men do and are trapped by the same glass ceilings that stifle white women's professional growth. They must also contend with on-the-job sexual harassment by both Black and white men, and they rarely bring home paychecks equal to either their Black male or white female counterparts. Yes, sometimes Black professional women do get bitter. Bitterness may be a logical reaction to the numbing realities of the corporate and professional world. But the bitter sister stereotype perverts what is a healthy anger at unfair treatment into a destructive, power-hungry, unbalanced caricature.

Many of us were far more likely to believe that Anita Hill, not Clarence Thomas, had a problem, because we are so very willing to accept the stereotype of Anita Hill as the bitter sister, angry at the world, and especially at the Black man who she thinks she's left behind.

The bitter sister stereotype tells others:

- Black women are never happy.
- Black women like to tear Black men down.
- Black women have nothing real to complain about.
- Black women who are professionally successful have no time for Black men.
- Black women are envious of Black men who are professionally successful.

The bitter sister stereotype tells Black women:

- Black women who complain are just asking for trouble.
- Black women should never call attention to their own problems or concerns if they will make a Black man look bad.
- If Black women pursue professional careers, they will find themselves estranged from Black men.

Neglectful Welfare Mothers

According to the news, they're everywhere. In Chicago, a group of five crack-addicted mothers is arrested for leaving their children in a filthy apartment; in South Carolina, pregnant drug users deliver their babies and are shackled to their beds the moment the children are born, arrested for child abuse. If you believe the news, Black mothers, especially young ones, are having children to get welfare benefits, and are beating, starving, and abandoning their unwanted children in projects and alleys all over the nation.

The neglectful (and/or abusive) welfare mother stereotype is a very new one, one that is actually in direct conflict with the mammy stereotype. Historically, if there was one thing Black women *could* do (besides work) it was raise children. Now we can't even manage that. Where did this new view of Black women come from? What's it all about?

As with all stereotypes, this one started with a kernel of truth that has been manipulated in many ways. The problem of drug use and addiction, especially the explosion of the crack trade, is very real. It has had a profound impact on African-American communities throughout the country. Yes, there are growing numbers of parents who are addicted and are unable to care for their children. Many of these parents are poor and on welfare. But what those who accept this stereotype fail to realize is that drug addiction and child neglect and abuse are national problems, not Black ones. We rarely see the children of other races who are left to fend for themselves by addicted parents, but they do exist. It is easier, however, to portray drug addiction and the havoc it wreaks on families as products of Black moral weakness than to address the realities of drug use as a pervasive aspect of American culture. It is also much simpler to blame the mothers of these neglected or abused children than it is to address the role of the fathers in the situation. The women are often scapegoated while the men escape all responsibility. Finally, this stereotype has at its core our failure to understand the causes and meanings of addiction, our own stereotypes of drug users, and the lack of proper treatment for those with drug problems. Rather than examine what would make a mother leave her children in squalor, with no heat or food, we simply label her an addict and toss her away.

The neglectful welfare mother stereotype tells others:

- Black women are lazy.
- Black women have more babies to collect welfare checks.
- Black women are sexually promiscuous.
- Black women don't know how to take care of their children.

The neglectful welfare mother stereotype tells Black women:

- Middle-class Black women are better than poor Black women. (Middle-class women know how to raise their children.)
- When we have trouble parenting, it is because of our own moral failings, not because of oppression, poverty, or addiction.
- Addiction is not a disease; it's a moral weakness.

So, if we accept the messages we get from popular culture, Black women are overweight mammies, uptight Sapphires, maladjusted tragic mulattos, hot-to-trot Jezebels, lonely bitter sisters, and hopeless addicts on welfare who can't even care for our children. Some choices! Who would want to be any of these? Fortunately, popular culture isn't the only place we learn about what it means to be a Black woman. But these messages are strong, and though we may not believe what they tell us about ourselves, our friends, coworkers, employers, landlords, partners, and even family members often do. Whether we accept any of these stereotypes or not, they undeniably influence how others view and interact with us, making it difficult for us to be our true selves and find the love, security, and peace we need. We know that this is unfair, and for some of us, this knowledge leads to hopelessness and despair. Survivors in the extreme, however, Black women have often reacted to these stereotypes of themselves by creating another, one that is empowering on the surface but ultimately just as damaging as the others: the superwoman. Who is the superwoman, and where do we learn about her? She is often the person to whom we are closest—our mother.

Mama Said: Lessons Learned at Home

If you were raised by your mother, chances are that she influenced your ideas about what it means to be a Black woman more than anyone else in your life. Other Black women—grandmothers, aunts, friends, teachers—may also have played a role, but mothers are the primary passers of the torch of Black womanhood.

Mothers teach their daughters about adult life primarily by example, although their words, whether tossed off casually or delivered in a carefully thought-out speech, can be equally influential. If a mother works and enjoys it, her daughter learns that work can be a fulfilling part of life. If she finds it drudgery, the daughter may grow up to think the same and look for someone to support her, or she may actively seek work that will make her happier than her mother's work made her. If a mother tells her daughter that she has to help to run the household, while she absolves her son of such responsibility, the daughter may grow up thinking it is a woman's duty to run a home and she should not expect help from men. If a mother constantly complains that men are no good, a daughter will probably grow up to feel the same way, at least until it is proven otherwise. And if a mother never complains, never breaks down or seems vulnerable, a daughter will learn to keep her complaints to herself. She will learn that women are invulnerable. No matter what a mother does, how she reacts, what she believes in, or what she says, she is her daughter's primary teacher. The daughter may learn to emulate, or she may learn to react in opposition, but either way, she learns from her mother's actions and attitudes.

So what do Black women learn from their mothers? For many of our mothers, Black womanhood meant two things: strength and pain. Get any five sisters in a room and at least four will tell stories of how their mothers worked all day (or all night), cooked and cleaned, raised several children, nurtured a man who was mistreated by the system, and was still full of praise on Sunday morning. Some will tell of mothers who supported children alone, making meals of beans and rice stretch for days; or mothers who were intimidated, threatened, or beaten by husbands or boyfriends; or mothers who routinely suffered humiliation at the hands of bosses at jobs they hated. And almost all of them will talk about their mother's strength. No matter what, they'll say, Mama kept on.

Of course, some Black women don't keep on. Some can't. But if there is one prevailing image we have of ourselves, it's that we can survive anything. We get that image from our mothers, who frequently shield us from the truth of their feelings. Our history in this country has taught Black women to be strong, to protect our families from racism and discrimination. Our mothers, therefore, teach us to be strong by pressing on. Black women don't have time to break down, they tell us. Even when our mothers cry, they often try to keep it from us. They pull themselves together quickly and tell us everything is all right. Our mothers are supposed to be superwomen, and that's what they teach us to be. These superwoman lessons start early and are reinforced throughout our lives.

Superwoman lesson #1: We are the mules of the world. What does it mean to be a mule of the world? For Nanny, the wise and weathered grandmother in *Their Eyes Were Watching God*, Zora Neale Hurston's classic tale of a Black woman's journey to self-discovery, being a mule of the world meant being both powerless and strong. As Nanny explains to her sheltered granddaughter, Janie, Black women are often the lowest on the totem pole:

> *Honey, de white man is de ruler of everything as fur as Ah been able tuh find out . . . So de white man throw down de load an tell de nigger man tuh pick it up. He pick it up because he have to, but he don't tote it. He hand it to his womenfolks. De nigger woman is de mule uh de world so fur as Ah can see.*

For Nanny, an ex-slave who escaped into the swamps of Florida with her week-old baby, being a mule meant working until your bones creaked, your skin split, and your face turned to leather from the hot sun in the fields, all without a grunt of complaint. It later meant running a white family's home and taking care of their kids. It meant being strong enough to endure rape by her master, whippings, humiliation, escape, raising a daughter (the product of that rape), losing a daughter (who fell apart after being raped herself, and ran away after Janie, the product of that rape, was born), and raising her abandoned granddaughter. In short, being a "mule of the world" meant—and means—taking it all and enduring. It means somehow reconciling the fact that our lives have little currency in the larger society with the fact that we are invaluable to those who depend on us.

Celeste learned superwoman lesson #1 from her mother, who always put the needs of others before her own. She describes the responsibilities of the modern-day Black superwoman, a role Celeste has been playing all her life.

> *My mother went without a lot of things because she had to put her needs aside—well, she chose to—in order to put our needs first or to get something that she felt was important for us. I think that women tend to do that. So, I don't think it's any surprise that I would invest in my husband, that I would look around and find somebody else to invest in other than myself. I don't think that we're taught to do that [invest in ourselves].*
>
> *I think part of it is a gender thing. It's funny how men can just come home, not all men, but a lot of men, could come home and not feel like they have any obligation in the house. Women are taught that they cook, and they've got to keep things clean. And men aren't taught that. So, a lot of men come home and it's like, freedom. You come home and it's another job.*
>
> *Women have a tendency to invest in other people. I think men do a better job of investing in themselves. I've seen men*

at work who come in and work is the number one thing with them. It's like their lives revolve around just them. And me, I've always had all these other people to worry about. I see these men and I just think, "Hey, they're so lucky to come to work and just be able to just do their work." I've got all these other worries that follow me around all the time. I never can shed one part of my life. And I'm not the only one. I see other women going out and trying to run their errands during lunch hour. And men, you don't see them running like down to the store to pick up something because they're not going to have time when they get home. They go off and they leisurely walk with their blazers over their shoulders off to lunch. And it's the women with their tennis shoes running around like crazy. Trying to do it all and coming home on the bus.

Being the mules of the world has created quite a bind for Black women. On the one hand, all that suffering and hardship *has* given us endurance and fortitude. It has helped us persevere in spite of the odds. Unfortunately, many of us call this strength. On the other hand, it has exacted a great psychological toll. As the Black feminist author bell hooks writes, ". . . to be strong in the face of oppression is not the same as overcoming oppression . . . endurance is not to be confused with transformation." African-American women are proud of our strength and ability to endure, but we must recognize that this strength has come at a price. That price is often our psychological health. Because we take pride in our ability to be strong and supportive, we can find it difficult to admit that we can't always bear up, that we are hurting, or that we need help. We have no problem being the shoulder for our partners, friends, and children to cry on, but we feel guilty or ashamed when we need a shoulder for ourselves.

Many Black women find it hard to admit they are overworked, overwhelmed, underloved, and depressed. After all, the mule never collapses under her load. She takes on the burden and continues, slowly and steadily, down the path. So instead of complaining or asking for help, many Black women try to keep on while they medicate their pain in self-destructive ways: by overeating, smoking, drinking, or using drugs. Others, like Celeste, just start working harder.

I had to be superwoman everywhere. I was trying to be superwoman at work. I was trying to be superwoman at home with a husband who was getting increasingly distant, irresponsible, immature. He needed mothering all the time. At the depth of my depression he quit his job and made me the sole wage earner at a time when I was dragging to work and really wanted to take six months off because of my emotional state. And he was totally against it. He told me that it was irresponsible. How could I do that? When the bills were paid he quit his job behind my back. And he later told me he quit when he did because he knew I was too helpless to do anything about it. So, I became not only somebody in need of a lot of support, but I had to provide financial support and emotional support. And it was just . . . it was overwhelming.

And after my honeymoon period [at work], three or four months, it's funny. I found out that a new manager was coming in. And I got this really sickening feeling that was really strange when I found out. I guess maybe it was just logic that had been telling me "things are going to be different," and things were. Everything that had been promised in this job evaporated. I was doing exactly the job that I feared I would. I didn't want to do it. I did all this agonizing taking this job and found myself really unhappy in it. I was getting depressed. At that time, I thought it was solely the job situation and my frustration there. And one of my personality traits is that I'm a real hard worker. I come from a family with a real strong work ethic. So, as I started getting depressed in this job, I started working harder. I worked longer hours. I became a super worker. And everyone's coming over to me going "You're producing more than anybody." People used to tease, "All we need is you. You can do it all by yourself." The more unhappy I was, the harder I worked. I was more frustrated that the job still wasn't what I wanted. And I really started to go down, down, down and started getting really depressed.

There is another message in superwoman lesson #1: that Black women should not expect too much out of life. Don't get hung up on your wants and dreams, because there is too much work to do, too many people to care for.

There are important things to be learned from superwoman lesson #1, among them the lesson that we are incredible women who embody the spirit of survival. But we must challenge the notion that we are the mules of the world who are willing and able to carry everyone's burden but unable to unburden ourselves, even when our lives depend on it.

Superwoman lesson #2: Mama duties don't stop at your front door. Our African-influenced extended-family tradition has helped us survive thus far. Though many researchers have maligned and misrepresented the Black family, we know that our willingness to extend ourselves for kin is one of our greatest strengths. Though you might not be able to rely on anyone else's help, relatives can often be counted on to take you in when you are down on your luck. They may even loan you money or help you find a job. We see helping our own as our duty. After all, if we don't look out for each other, who will?

For some Black women, however, this willingness to help family members in need gets translated into a sense of responsibility to others—whether immediate family, extended family, friends, or community—that can be self-destructive. Such women feel they must take care of everyone, but they neglect to take care of themselves or their primary relationships. These Black superwomen offer their homes, their time, and their energy to anyone who appears to need it, often at their own expense.

Celeste learned superwoman lesson #2 from her mother, whose concern for relatives seemed to get in the way of her most important relationships.

> *My mother was always helping relatives. We had a cousin who came up here and moved in with my parents. My mother heard that she couldn't get a job in the South, so she brought her up here and helped her get a job and get established. This cousin was a very difficult person. She almost seemed to have the desire to break my parents up. She really caused a lot of conflict in the house. But my mother is always helping people, always bringing somebody in.*

Her mother's always-take-care-of-your-own point of view has made Celeste feel a sense of responsibility to family and to other African Americans who may be in need of help. While she thinks this feeling of extended kinship is a positive and necessary thing, she also wonders if we might sometimes put too much pressure on ourselves to lift as we climb.

> *I do feel that it's important for me to help others because I'm a professional person. I could give something back. I feel strongly about that. But Black people are always having to shoulder burdens like that. We've got to lift all the people up. And I don't think everybody can do that or should be expected to do that. Certain people who want to and have the means to, should. But I know right now I have to make a difference in my own life. I haven't been attending to any of my needs and I've realized that.*

Superwoman lesson #3: What's (self-) love got to do with it? In her 1973 novel, *Sula*, author Toni Morrison heartbreakingly portrays the mother-daughter relationship between Eva Peace and her daughter, Hannah. When Hannah asked her mother if she had ever loved her children, Eva's reply was not what Hannah expected:

> . . . *You settin' here with your healthy-ass self and ax me did I love you? Them big old eyes in your head would a been two holes full of maggots if I hadn't. . . . With you all coughin' and me watchin' so TB wouldn't take you off and if you was sleepin' quiet I thought, O Lord, they dead and put my hand over your mouth to feel if the breath was comin' what you talkin' bout did I love you girl I stayed alive for you can't you get that through your thick head or what is between your ears, heifer?*

For Eva, and for many Black mothers of previous generations, loving your children meant staying alive for them, and keeping them alive. Love meant survival. There wasn't time for much more than that.

The same was true of teaching your children to feel good about themselves. It has been, for most of our years on American soil, much more important for Black children to learn their place than to feel good about themselves. Little Black boys who did not know their place might end up hanging from a poplar tree; their sisters might be raped. (Some in this country still operate under the assumption that Blacks should know their place; think about what happened to Rodney King).

But survival is no longer enough. Many of us have no problem taking care of our basic survival needs. Once those needs are met, we still feel that something is missing. That something is self-love and self-esteem. It is recognizing the need to spend time on ourselves and with ourselves. Seattle psychotherapist Julia A. Boyd, in her book *In the Company of My Sisters: Black Women and Self-Esteem*, explains that although self-esteem was not an issue for these generations of Black mothers because the realities of life could not allow it to be, it is an issue for Black women today.

> The concept of loving one's self was a foreign concept to my parents, because it was a foreign concept to their parents. I once heard a great teacher say, you can teach others only to the extent of your own knowledge; in this regard my parents gave to me what had been given to them. The unfortunate news is that the traditional ethnic structure that helped my parents survive their lives and sustained me through childhood falls short of what I need in today's world as a mature adult.

Many of us simply were not given the tools to love ourselves. Other important tools were passed on: how to work, how to raise children so they don't get killed, how to take care of a man who the rest of the world treats like a child, and how to get by on your own. Our parents showed their love through these lessons and through providing for our physical and material needs (and that was often hard enough). Superwoman lesson #3 is simple: Black women have too much to do—and too much to worry about—to get hung up on loving themselves.

The superwoman stereotype is dangerous because it tells us that we can take anything anyone throws our way. We need little nurturing or support. We will adjust just fine. It tells us we can't break down or fall apart, so when we (inevitably) do, we feel we have failed ourselves, our families, even the entire race.

We need to give ourselves a break. Black women must come to understand (and must make others understand) that we are not superwomen, that there is no shame in not being able to hold up all the time. We must stop accepting the fact that life is hard for Black women. We must start challenging, instead. We will receive better treatment only when we demand it, and in order to demand it, we must first believe that we deserve it.

3

. . . .

Living in the Integration Generation: Race, Stress, and Depression

Optimism was high in the late 1950s and 1960s. The civil rights movement brought the promise of a new society, one in which all people, no matter what their race or color, would have the opportunity to live the American Dream. As Dr. Martin Luther King, Jr., said so eloquently, we would see a day when we were judged not by the color of our skin, but by the content of our character.

Indeed, much has changed since the days of the marches and sit-ins. Separate rest rooms and water fountains are dim memories, and may even seem unbelievable to the youngest of us. Affirmative action has led to increased opportunities in America's colleges and corporations, which has in turn swelled the ranks of the Black middle class. Blacks and whites can, and often do, socialize, date, and marry freely. Yet there is still a palpable sense of disappointment, even betrayal, among even the most seemingly well-off African Americans. In his book *The Rage of a Privileged Class*, journalist Ellis Cose sums up the feelings of many Blacks who have, on the surface, made it:

> *Despite its very evident prosperity, much of America's Black middle class is in excruciating pain. And that distress— although most of the country does not see it—illuminates a*

serious American problem: the problem of the broken cove-
nant, of the pact ensuring that if you work hard, get a good
education, and play by the rules, you will be allowed to ad-
vance and achieve to the limits of your ability.

Cose goes on to illustrate case after case in which this cov-
enant has been broken. Each of the brothers and sisters he
interviewed told the same story: that despite their intelligence,
hard work, dedication, and skill, they still faced racism and
discrimination in school and on the job. Their advancement
and opportunities were limited because of it. All of them were
angry. Many were also depressed.

While such prejudice is obviously bad for business—and for
the well-being of the society at large—it has a tremendous effect on the psyches of those who experience it. Normal job- or
school-related stress, combined with stress caused by discrimination and racism, can be overwhelming. Add to this the feeling of having been betrayed by a system whose rules one has
followed, and depression can often be the result.

Also troubling is the fact that Blacks who find themselves in
such situations rarely get the support they need to get through
them. Friends and family members (especially those who have
not worked or gone to school in similar environments) may
not be able to relate to their problems. Coworkers and super-
visors may think Blacks who complain of discrimination are
crybabies or troublemakers, making the work environment
even more tense. Other Blacks on the job or at school may see
each other as competition, and may not trust each other
enough to see any common interest. This leaves many of us
alone with our stress, anger, and frustration.

The Broken Covenant:
Celeste, Latrice, and Maya

Celeste, like many Black women, was raised to believe in the
redemptive nature of hard work. Though her parents had not

gone to college, they expected her to do so. When an opportunity came along for Celeste to attend a private college-preparatory school, her parents, particularly her mother, thought it was a chance of a lifetime.

I went to an all-white boarding school. I was the first Black student. I was treated like crap. It was very difficult because my family is a very working-class family. I look back now and I guess we were even poor at times, although I never thought about it. I always got what I wanted. We always had nice clothes to wear to church on Sunday.

Then all of a sudden I went to this boarding school and it was like we had nothing. I went to school with these kids who were talking, "For my sixteenth birthday, I got a wing in the house." It didn't compute with me. I thought, "What does this mean? Does this mean that something is wrong with us; that we are inferior people or something? That here my parents are working hard and we have this little shoe box house, and these people are getting wings to the house for their birthday?" . . . It was this whole other world.

These people had never been around Black people, except as servants. So, there was a lot of racism. They told jokes. Certain people wouldn't associate themselves with me. They let it be known that they didn't befriend niggers. Some people didn't say anything. They just gave me the cold shoulder all the time.

I remember one thing that was really painful. I was among this group of friends. I wondered why this girl was always quiet when I was around. And finally, one day, somebody told me, "You ought to stop hanging around Marcia because she hates Black people. As soon as you walk out, she starts telling nigger jokes." And of course, all the rest of my friends were with her all the time. There were a lot of things like that.

There was a lot of stress during that time between me and my mother. My mother would have liked to have gone to college, but she didn't have the opportunity. A boarding school was a real dream for her. She was very much into education and getting this type of opportunity. So, any grief that I expressed wasn't appreciated. And I understand it now. I've certainly forgiven her and I love my mother and everything. But it was very hard because I didn't have any emotional support at the time. There was no one to turn to. Dealing with my own self-esteem as a Black woman in this all-white, very privileged environment where I was getting messages all the time: I'll never be good enough; I'm not the same; I'm not part of the group; I'll never be one of you. . . . I have nightmares about that experience to this day. It wasn't all horrible, but it was very difficult.

Celeste felt completely alone, both at home and at school. The extreme class differences and the racism at school kept her from getting really close to any of her peers during her teen years—a time in life when making friends and separating from parents is very important. And her mother, who no doubt thought she was doing the best thing for her daughter by sending her to an exclusive boarding school, could not see that Celeste was extremely unhappy there. Consequently, Celeste felt uncomfortable in both places.

I would go home most weekends. Starting Thursday night, I would get really tense about going home, because my mother just didn't understand. And I would be tense all weekend, knowing that I was going to have to go back to school.

Celeste's first bouts with depression came during this very stressful, very lonely time.

> *I would feel horrible. Then I would say, "Well, next week
> will be better." But it was the same week after week, month
> after month, finally year after year. And so, while before I
> might have a couple of down days, now I would feel really
> down. But I always came out of it. I always felt better.*

Celeste was able to emerge from these depressive episodes
on her own. But looking back, they seem to have been a warning of more serious depressions to come. Unfortunately, the
stresses in Celeste's academic and professional lives were just
beginning. As these stresses got worse, so did her depression.
One New Year's Eve was particularly bad:

> *I got some whiskey, mixed it with 7UP, and drank myself
> into unconsciousness. I literally blacked out. I hated it
> [drinking]. I don't think I had drunk anything before. I
> woke up several times during the night and I would just
> black out again, vomiting all over myself. I remember think-
> ing, "I'm going to just feel good this New Year's Eve. I'm
> going to drink this and I'm going to get drunk and I'm going
> to feel good. And I don't care about anything else."*

Celeste toughed it out at the boarding school for four years.
While she does feel she got a good academic preparation for
college there, she is well aware of the emotional toll taken by
four years of isolation and lack of support. Celeste attended a
predominantly white college, but was fortunate enough to live
on an all-Black floor in her freshman dorm, where she found
friendship with people who could understand her experience.
College did present other problems for Celeste, as we will see
later, but having other Blacks around served as a buffer between Celeste and a sometimes hostile, often indifferent white
environment.

Faced with racism and little support again in graduate

school and later, on the job, Celeste began to feel the anger and betrayal Cose describes in his book:

> *I have felt the sting of racism many times. When I was in graduate school, doors were literally slammed in my face. I remember a white male student coming over to me in a class where I was the only Black student and starting to moan and whine about how much work we had to do and how he didn't get it finished and it was just too much to do and nobody can do all of that and "Did you do it?" And I said, "Yeah, I did it." And he got up and never spoke another word to me. He came to me because I was the Black person in class. . . . I had to be the dumbest one there, I could not have done [the assignment].*
>
> *It's like race is an issue all the time. I've always believed that if you work hard enough, then you are supposed to be able to overcome or work your way through certain things. But people break the rules all the time. And I'm wondering why they aren't playing fair. That kind of feeling contributed to my depression. It's like I'm playing by the rules, but nobody else seems to be. I'm being honest and I'm working hard, and everybody else is lying and cheating and being racist. . . . Why doesn't everybody else follow these rules? It's like it's some kind of cruel unfairness.*

Celeste's experiences of racism, classism, and isolation were anything but subtle. They left her with a feeling that the world is fundamentally unfair, that no matter how hard you work, you may never be allowed to achieve to the limits of your capability. These feelings undoubtedly trigger and feed Celeste's depressive episodes.

While the kinds of discrimination Celeste dealt with are by no means unheard of, the less obvious insults common to Latrice's experience are now more likely than outright racism. The cumulative effect of these smaller slights, snubs, and oversights can be just as painful as the effects of more overt prejudice and racism. In Latrice's case, they have contributed to her depression.

Latrice had been putting in a lot of hard work and extra hours at the women's clothing store where she worked. In her first six months, she had learned everything she needed to know for her position and had mastered her boss's job. She even volunteered to take on extra work:

> I basically ran the store. My manager was late every morning. And by the time she got to work, I'd already started doing the daily receipts, got the inventory done, had my ordering together, and was on my way to the bank. And I felt I did a damn good job running her store. I did it because I was ambitious, because I wanted something, so I worked hard for it.

It soon became clear, however, that Latrice was not going to reap the benefits of her hard work.

> [The manager] brought a new coworker in and I helped train this girl. Then, when the assistant manager left, my manager hired this other girl to be her assistant manager. This girl didn't know a thing about ordering, about managing the floor, how to take the registers down. It bugged me. Because, yes, the woman was white. I was very pissed off that I worked fourteen hours a day on a job that was only supposed to be eight. I trained this woman. And what really unnerved me was that I had been totally loyal to my manager and I felt like an idiot for this.
>
> When I didn't get hired as assistant manager, my manager was too much of a wimp to tell me herself. She had the district manager come to our store. When he told me, I could not help it. I got emotional. They told me that the reason I could not be assistant manager was because I wanted what

*I wanted when I wanted it. And I'm thinking, "If you
worked fourteen hours a day and you did all this crap, and
you trained somebody, too, you'd want what you wanted
when you wanted it as well. And I'm sure you would not
want to do a manager's job and not get paid what the manager was getting paid." I thought that was the most absurd
thing they could possibly tell me as a reason as to why I did
not get a position that I worked damn hard to get.*

Like Celeste, Latrice got little support from her family. Her
mother, who was raised at a time when Blacks who made waves
could be putting themselves in serious danger, offered advice
that Latrice found out of date.

*When I talked to my mother about it, she said, "Well, you
have to play the game by other people's rules until you have
your own game board." And I'm thinking that's bull———.
You know, if you want something, you've got to go out there
and get it, but you can't be slighted and just accept it. You
can't accept people just mistreating you because they feel
that's what they can do.*

Rejecting her mother's advice, Latrice handled things her
own way. In retrospect, she realizes her rash actions made
things even worse.

*So then I got pissed off. I called the main office and told
them, "Look, you all got to transfer me out of this store. I
don't care where you send me, just get me out of this store."
So, they sent me to fifty miles from my house. It was like,
"We're going to teach you." I got so depressed up there [at
the new store]. I used to have crying spells on the way to
work. Because I couldn't believe how this store had mistreated
me after I was doing all this work.*

Depressed and angry, Latrice soon gave up.

> *From that point on, it was like, "You all ain't playin' fair. I'm trying to play fair. I can't be out here like this having you all walk all over me."*

Because of her depression, Latrice's performance at work slipped considerably. Many days, she could find no reason to get up and go to work, so she called in sick. When she did go, she arrived late, and she was lethargic and distant—not exactly the best attitude for someone who has to wait on customers. She wasn't surprised when she lost her job, and she jumped at a cousin's suggestion that Latrice take a job at the bank where she worked.

> *When they fired me, it felt like a burden had been lifted off my shoulders. I really did not want to be there and they weren't treating me the way I felt I should be treated. I kind of got the screw-you attitude. But once I left and got this other funky job at a bank, I felt like I had made the wrong decision, like maybe I should have let them walk across my back just a little bit more, you know.*

The new job only worsened Latrice's depression. She had no interest in what she was doing, but felt she had to stay because her cousin had helped her get the job. She had little energy to look for another job; the depression had settled in and the most minor tasks seemed overwhelming. Latrice began to wonder if she would ever realize her dreams. She doubted her talents, her ability, and her ambition. Though she had always been proud of the fact that she wanted to make the most of her life, she now wondered if the stress of going up against discrimination and dealing with company politics was worth it. The thought of fighting losing battles the rest of her work life didn't appeal to Latrice, but the thought of giving up on her goals made her feel like a failure. She knows she could let go of her dreams and try to find fulfillment through having children—something many of her friends have done. But she has always wanted something else from her life. When we met Latrice, she was still struggling with these feelings.

> *If I wasn't ambitious and I wasn't striving for anything, then where I am now would be OK. Since I have ambition, it kind of bugs me out that I am striving for something and I don't have it. It's like you're constantly trying to move this mountain and you're always being told there's some reason that you can't do what you want to do.*
>
> *I'm also seeing brothers and sisters who are like, "Look, this mountain can move, and you've got to push it. Let me show you how to do it." And those people are the most stressed out. It's like the people who actually are ambitious, who are actually getting up there every day and trying to live their lives on their own terms, are the ones who are always stressed out. The ones who I hang out with the most, who are just kickin' back, you know, taking life as it comes, are the least stressed people. I want to be stress free, but I also want to be the person that I think that God intended for me to be. But sometimes when it gets tough, it's like, "Man, forget this. I should just have a baby."*

Like Celeste, Latrice had expected that playing by the rules would help her get to where she wanted to be. She didn't expect the rules to be unfair or that they would change halfway through the game. Though her mother told her she had to accept the patently unfair rules until she had her own game board, Latrice had a hard time accepting this. For an intelligent, ambitious woman like Latrice, accepting unfairness meant accepting defeat—and depression. Latrice struggles against her depression daily, fighting the urge to give up on her dreams and just have a baby. When she is very depressed, these feelings of powerlessness against an unfair system often lead her to self-medicate with marijuana and overeating. Latrice's struggle with depression parallels her struggle to realize her ambitions.

Perhaps the most disturbing thing that Latrice alludes to is the fact that often, Blacks with the most ambition are also the most stressed out—and the most vulnerable to depression.

Maya has also found her dreams deferred and her depression exacerbated by discrimination and petty office politics. Maya is a clerical worker in a state bureaucracy, where the extremely politicized environment determines how far you will advance, no matter how long you have worked there or how qualified you may be. She wonders if the overt racism her mother and grandmother faced might not have been easier to handle than the insidious prejudice she encounters on the job:

> *The issues that my mother and grandmother faced, at least they faced them from people who actually said to them, "You are a nigger." What I get is, "Well, I'm sorry, you can't be promoted because you need a degree. . . . Well, you have three and a half years of college. . . . Sorry, you need that last half year of college in order to get this promotion." It doesn't matter that you have ten years of experience and we are hiring people with cooking degrees and veterinarian degrees who are one or two years out of college. They have a degree.*

The racial hierarchy at Maya's job is very clear, and movement into the higher ranks is strictly regulated.

> *I could name how many white clerks there are. It's not so much that they are all Black, but the great majority are Hispanic, Black, and the third down the list is Asian. I can count three white clerks in our office, out of a total of sixty-five. Now, if you want to see that ratio get flipped upside*

*down, I can tell you how many Black, Indian, Asian, and
Hispanic people are in the managerial offices. I just named
them all, there is one of each; there's four.*

In her ten-year tenure, Maya has applied for other jobs in
her department many times, only to be rebuffed because of
her lack of a college degree. Though the state does provide a
tuition reimbursement plan, it only covers classes at the local
community colleges, which do not grant four-year degrees.
Without tuition assistance, Maya has found it difficult to finish
school.

As often happens when a large number of workers vie for a
few promotions, employees at Maya's workplace do not trust
each other, and Maya feels as if she is always watching her back.
This combined stress eventually made her physically ill and depressed.

*I began having migraine headaches. I had so much stress
on my system that I started getting constant colds and flu
and all sorts of upper respiratory infections. I was depressed
tremendously and noticeably—it was interfering with my being able to do anything else outside of that office. I also slept
a great deal.*

*The environment there is so incredibly stressful and hor-
rible and people are so casually cruel to the clerks. It does
not help that the clerks then are like crabs in a barrel. If one
of us goes up [to a supervisor] and says, "Look, you've got
to cut this stuff out" and then we have some success, immediately people start clawing at you and talking about
you—we're pulling each other down. So, you're talking about
a pressure cooker every single day. All of that stress from the
job produced my physical symptoms, until I had a fever that
was so high that my pancreas finally broke down [leading
to insulin-dependent diabetes]. In seven days I lost twenty-
one pounds.*

Her physical illnesses (which, in addition to diabetes and migraines, include irritable bowel syndrome, another condition easily worsened by stress) and her depression have made it difficult for Maya to consider leaving her job. Working for a large government bureaucracy does have some advantages, and one of these is excellent health insurance. Maya fears—rightly so—that she will not be able to find comparable coverage in a smaller or private-sector setting. Even if she did find a job with good health insurance, her preexisting conditions—those she actually needs treatment for—probably wouldn't be covered.

Unlike Celeste and Latrice, Maya has not always felt alone in her predicament. She had many friends who dealt with similar problems on the job.

> I hung out with a big crowd of friends . . . and all of us were bitching and complaining about work. There wasn't one of us who didn't say, "God, I can't believe you. What do you mean? No, they didn't do that."
>
> We all did different kinds of work. There were even those of us who were professionals. I have a friend who has a master's degree in literature, and she is teaching at a college now. She's been there for going on four years now and even her with a master's degree, she is still dealing with the same crap. Another friend of ours, Greg, is working for a family-owned manufacturing company. It took seven years before he was promoted or offered a raise.

Maya took a proactive stance to combat her job woes: she became a union organizer. While this has made her feel as if she and the other clerks have a little more power on the job, it has also produced more stress. Long contract negotiations and bitter fights with management take a lot out of her. What's more, her union work has made her quite unpopular with management, making a promotion even less likely. This has led her to exhibit some passive-aggressive behavior:

> *It has been a source of much satisfaction to me that I can*
> *formally, in front of their faces and everybody else's faces,*
> *push my bosses around now, because I can say, "Oh, you*
> *have that concern? Well, wait, let me call up the union."*
> *. . . It's very satisfying. So, yeah, it has brought some per-*
> *sonal satisfaction.*

But even this slight satisfaction does not overcome the depression that has enveloped Maya's life. While Maya has been depressed most of her life, her job situation certainly contributes to her chronically depressed state.

> *You get saturated in depression because there are all these*
> *circumstances surrounding you. . . . No matter where you*
> *turn, if you find yourself lifting up a little bit, then you get*
> *this big gloop of just horrible stuff going on around you. It*
> *may not even be directly aimed at you, but it is going on*
> *around you and it makes you feel terrible.*

Racism, discrimination, and prejudice are powerful stressors, but they are not the only problems Black women may face at school or on the job. Even sisters who work in relatively enlightened settings (or even all-Black ones) face on-the-job stress; and sisters who find solid Black communities in college or go to historically Black universities deal with other, very real stresses, too. Heavy workloads, juggling work and school or work and family, falling out with friends or coworkers—all these can trigger or exacerbate depressions in people who are vulnerable to them.

Keisha had been depressed throughout her teen years, and the stress of college life pushed her into the most severe depression she had experienced to that point. The depression was precipitated by a breakup with a boyfriend, but worsened under the weight of schoolwork and decisions about her future:

That semester I decided I didn't want to go to medical school.
I went to Dawn [her sister, a medical resident at the time]
who was in the hospital for thirty-six hours on call, and told
her I didn't want to go to medical school. At the time I was
pre-med. I was in physics and I thought, "This is so hard."
I was just really crying all the time. I felt like a failure,
like I had failed my family because they wanted another
doctor. I barely made it through that semester.

Keisha went home for the summer, hoping that being away from school would help her depression. It didn't, and Keisha and her family soon realized she needed treatment.

Elaine isn't sure whether her first severe depressive episode was triggered by job stress or if personality changes brought about by the depression actually heightened her stress level. Either way, she knows that her unhappiness at work led her to a rash decision: retiring on the spur of the moment.

A teacher for twenty-four years, Elaine had always gotten along very well with her coworkers. Of course, there had been people she was not so fond of, but she was the kind of person who could be civil, even friendly, to anybody. She felt it part of her role as a professional to treat all her coworkers with respect.

Lately, though, she had become increasingly irritated by the political maneuverings of the parent-run local school council and some of the teachers at the school. Elaine felt that this group was unfairly criticizing the school principal for political—and racial—reasons: the principal was white; the local school council, the teachers in question, and the students were Black. The teachers and the council president wanted to replace the white principal with a Black man. But Elaine, who had worked directly under the principal for many years, did not support this plan. She soon found herself outcast. Other teachers stopped cooperating with her. One even falsely accused Elaine of slamming a door in her face. The atmosphere in the school became extremely tense. Hurt by accusations that she was an Uncle Tom and frustrated by the lack of cooperation from the other teachers, Elaine abruptly transferred from the school she had been in for over ten years. She ended up in a Hispanic school and felt overwhelmed because she knew very little about Hispanic cultures and spoke no Spanish. After taking a week sick leave, Elaine called in her retirement. A few weeks later, considering suicide, she called her parish priest, who convinced her to go to the hospital.

Don't Let It Bring You Down: Handling Race-Related Stress

No matter how much progress we make, it always seems that someone, at some level, is questioning us. Whites often question our intelligence and our ability to do our jobs. Some un-reconstructed racists still question our humanity. As Elaine learned, other Blacks may even question our commitment to the race if we do not go along with their way of thinking. Over time, all this questioning becomes another heavy burden, one that, when combined with all the other stresses of our lives, becomes very hard to bear.

Although great strides have been made, racism is still prevalent in the workforce and on college campuses. In some places, it is still overt and in-your-face. In most settings, however, racism has become much more subtle. Since it is now illegal to come right out and say things like "We'd rather not hire or promote Blacks," or "We don't want Blacks in our school," schools and workplaces have become far more creative in their excuses for bypassing us. One way of doing this is to make us feel personally inadequate. We are told we haven't paid our dues by bosses who have no intention of letting us pay them, or we hear we don't have the right credentials while others without those credentials advance anyway. We are assumed to belong in remedial classes, and are underrecruited at elite insitutions. We are often left, like Celeste, Maya, and Latrice, angry and unsupported, with nothing to do with that anger but let it eat away at us.

What's worse, we often fail to find support when we look for it. Traditionally, we would look to elders or mentors for advice. But many of us work in settings where we are one of only a handful of Blacks. Mentors are often nonexistent. Because of social changes, many elders in the community can't relate to our integration-generation dilemmas and therefore can't give useful advice. And, in a climate of fear, other Blacks on the job are likely to be more concerned with watching their backs than with supporting each other.

The situation in many schools is no better. Black students in predominantly white schools rarely have Black faculty members to call on for support and counsel. Those few existing Black mentors are usually so stressed by the demands of their jobs (and by having to prove themselves, as well) that they may not have much to give to students. Even those who try are sometimes overwhelmed by the needs of the Black students who rely on them.

Racism and discrimination are likely to be with us for some time to come. The challenge is how to maintain a sense of hope in the face of these destructive forces. Sometimes the answer is a political one, as in Maya's case. Becoming active in her union has at least given Maya an outlet for her anger, even though true change has been slow in coming. For others, who find the stresses of racism and discrimination unbearable, finding another job or transferring to another school might be the most viable option.

Support is key. Black professional groups can be lifelines, and almost every profession has one. Organizations like the National Black MBA Association, the National Medical Association, and the National Association of Black Journalists have local chapters in most major cities. Becoming active in such groups gives many Black professional women a safe space to talk about job-related pressures and stresses that they might not be able to discuss at work. Unions often have Black (or minority) caucuses that handle issues of discrimination and provide members the same kinds of opportunities for networking and support that professional organizations do. Black student organizations are invaluable for many Black students at mostly white schools. Take advantage of whatever support is available to you.

Psychotherapy can also be of great help in handling work- and school-related stresses. Many Black women (and men) find that therapy helps them develop a more healthy perspective on work and its attendant problems. Some therapists can teach you specific anger-management and stress-reduction techniques. A therapist may also be able to help you come up with strategies for combating and confronting racism on the job or at school. (See chapter 8 for information on types of psychotherapy and finding a therapist).

We do not have to be alone with our stress and anger. We do not have to be destroyed by it, either.

4

· · · · · · ·

Love Don't Love Nobody:
Self-Esteem, Relationships,
and Depression

Everybody needs love. We need to be loved by our parents and friends, boyfriends and girlfriends, husbands and wives. Without love, humans simply can't survive. Infants who are not loved and touched develop failure to thrive and can die within months, even though they may have been perfectly healthy at birth. Throughout life, we all search for the sense of attachment, fulfillment, and peace that comes from truly loving another person (and truly being loved).

Relationships are at the core of human experience. We are social, and no one can be healthy and exist completely apart from others. In her book *Silencing the Self: Women and Depression,* psychologist Dana Crowley Jack describes this relational theory of the self and depression:

> *From the relational viewpoint, the self (in both women and men) is part of a fundamentally social experience . . . the attainment of a sense of basic human connectedness is the goal of development. . . . If relatedness with others is of primary importance, it becomes clear why a person will go to any lengths, including altering the self, to establish and maintain intimate ties. From the relational perspective, depression is* interpersonal *[emphasis hers].*

Women, especially, define ourselves and our roles in relationship to others. We are mothers, daughters, sisters, lovers, and wives. We are socialized to be caretakers, nurturers, and peacemakers. Much of our self-esteem is tied to having what Jack calls "positive attachments"—in other words, healthy relationships, ones that help us grow. According to Jack, a woman's sense of self is directly related to how people in her life and society at large relate to her:

> *A woman forms images of self. . . . that directly reflect her interpersonal experiences—as able to give and receive love, or as unable; as worthy of care and support from others, or as unworthy; as free to be herself while maintaining connection, or as unfree. Because women's core sense of self is more relationally based than men's . . . then the qualities of current relationships—not just the relationships experienced in early childhood—may more deeply influence the female than the male self. . . . A woman's social context, both in particular relationships and in the wider world, fundamentally affects these images of self . . . According to the relational point of view, depression arises from the inability to make or sustain supportive, authentic connection with a loved person.*

Jack goes on to explain that while most psychological theory holds that depression is the result of the loss of another (like the loss of a lover or the death of a parent, especially a dominant one), she has found, by listening to women tell their stories of depression, that depressed women often experience a loss of themselves in a relationship. It is this loss of self, not simply a loss of relationship, that leads to depression. A loss of self can be described as a loss of self-esteem, a loss of agency (the ability to be self-determining), and a loss of voice. Celeste's story illustrates this loss of voice well. Though she was terribly unhappy in boarding school, she was not able to make her mother understand this because her voice was simply not heard, valued, and responded to. Celeste's voice was lost to her mother's, as were her needs and wishes.

In unhealthy relationships, women develop negative (or unproductive) senses of self, and negative, unproductive self-images are reinforced. As Jack points out, we develop views of ourselves as lovable or unlovable, as able to give and receive love or as unable, as a result of our interactions with others and the messages we get from society. So when those we are close to mistreat, abuse, ignore, belittle, or betray us, we may get the message that we deserve this treatment, that we somehow brought it on ourselves—especially if we have always been treated this way (or if we saw our mothers treated this way). Poor treatment by the ones we love sets us up to expect and accept continuing poor treatment, and this destroys our self-esteem. Without self-love and self-esteem, finding and accepting honest, mutual love is very hard to do.

Low self-esteem and feelings of worthlessness are two of the most pervasive symptoms of depression. Most depressed people, while in the depths of the illness, feel unloved and unlovable, as if their lives have no value whatsoever. They can't find anything good to say about themselves, and blame themselves for all their problems (even those that are clearly not their fault). They often blame themselves for other people's problems as well.

In addition to being a prevalent symptom of depression, low self-esteem is also a major risk factor for depression. This is because having low self-esteem makes us expect and accept less from life. Black women with low self-esteem don't think they deserve happiness, so they don't seek it out and they usually don't find it. They may think they don't deserve friends who care about them, or that people who are nurturing and loving would never be attracted to them. As a result, they may have difficulty finding caring, nurturing friends, or they may have a hard time relating to them. This is especially true of romantic relationships. Sisters with low self-esteem often have trouble finding relationships in which they are valued because they do not value themselves. They may be resigned to accept treatment that more self-confident and self-loving sisters would not put up with because they don't think they can do any better.

Low self-esteem engenders a vicious cycle: Having low self-esteem makes it hard to find and form good relationships; bad relationships further damage your self-esteem. Getting caught in this cycle can lead to depression, but for a sister who is already suffering from depression, this kind of relationship cycle can lead to the brink of suicide.

Why Do Some Black Women Have Low Self-Esteem?

Good self-esteem starts in childhood. Children don't come into this world knowing that their lives are valuable. They must be taught this through love, attention, nurturing, and discipline. Black children especially need to know that they are loved and cherished, because American society still tells them that their lives are worth less than those of their white peers. And Black girls, faced with the double constraints of racism and sexism, must understand that Blackness and being female are valuable.

But think back to chapter 2. Think of all the negative messages Black women get each day. Turn on the news: how many Black women are being accused of leaving their children at home alone while they go out to get high? How many politicians are chanting "Work, not welfare" while pictures of Black mothers flash in the background? Listen to the radio: How many raps drive home the assertion that we ain't nothin' but bitches and hos? How often do you hear a soulful voice singing "Baby I respect you"? How often do you hear "I want your sex"?

You may be thinking, "Yeah, that's true. But that stuff is just entertainment. It doesn't have anything to do with how I feel about myself." If you had a strong sense of self to begin with, it probably doesn't. You may be able to ignore it, or it may make you angry enough to write a letter to your local TV or radio station. But if you are already prone to believe, because of your experience, that Black women *are* the stereotypes, these messages may reaffirm what you already think about yourself and other Black women. (Of course, as we discussed in chapter 2, even if you don't believe what these messages say about Black women, they certainly shape how others view us. This limits our opportunities and affects our interactions with others in a very real way.)

How Does Low Self-Esteem Affect Our Relationships?

Black women with low self-esteem often find that their feelings about themselves affect their relationships in several ways:

- Low self-esteem makes Black women feel that they must *earn* the love of others. For these women, there is no such thing as unconditional love.
- Low self-esteem makes Black women equate *need* with *love*; when others need them, they feel loved. All of us need to feel needed. Knowing others rely on you makes you feel valuable. But being needed is only one part of being loved. The two are not the same.
- Low self-esteem leads Black women to accept treatment they don't deserve. They may think there is nothing better out there for them, or that they have brought the bad treatment on themselves. They may equate leaving a bad or unfulfilling relationship with personal failure. Leaving means you didn't try hard enough.
- Low self-esteem makes Black women think they need a

man to be complete. Women who think this way are not happy unless they are in a relationship. This kind of thinking leads some women to take what they can get—at any cost. They reason that any man is better than no man at all.

Celeste: A Need to Be Needed

Celeste's story illustrates all of these points. As you'll recall, Celeste had battled depression throughout her teen years. Four years of boarding school in a prestigious but hostile, all-white environment had battered her self-esteem. Her mother's inability to support her left Celeste feeling alone and vulnerable. College was an exciting opportunity; for the first time, Celeste felt she fit in. The young sisters and brothers she lived with on the all-Black floor of her dorm became a kind of surrogate family. And she found romance. Jason and Celeste connected immediately. Celeste felt he needed her, and feeling needed made her feel good.

> *Jason came from a troubled family, and I felt like I was going to help him. I was going to rescue him. He was so needy. He had no money, so I would take money that I had from my parents and buy him clothes, because he was really tall and gangly and his clothes never fit. I would buy books, school books for him. I took care of him, you know, in a motherly way.*

As time went on, Jason got very comfortable with being mothered by Celeste. They married a few years out of college, and throughout their marriage Celeste gave and gave, but got very little in return. It took a long time for her to realize this, however, because she felt needed. And if there is one thing Black women are taught, it is that our self-worth is tied to how much we give to others. Good sisters are those who can put the needs of others—their husbands, their children, their parents, and their community—before their own.

> *I now realize that I was attracted . . . to the fact that there was somebody there that would need me. That I could help him. I was helping him academically. I was helping him financially. I was getting something out of it, I guess, at that time. It was nice to feel needed and as if I was making a difference.*

Jason began to take advantage of Celeste. He expected her to be the adult in the relationship, while he indulged his whims. Because she did not believe in divorce (her Catholic faith frowned upon it), and because she still felt Jason needed her, Celeste put up with increasingly outrageous (and sometimes abusive) behavior. Looking back on their relationship, Celeste can now see how her need to be needed and her low self-esteem led her to accept substandard treatment.

> *I now see that my ex-husband and I should never have married, or that I should have ended that relationship a long time ago; that he had done a lot of things over the years that were intolerable and I put up with it . . . from his hitting me early in our relationship to him quitting jobs, being fired from jobs. He had never pulled his weight financially. I was always the hustler and he was out doing his thing.*
>
> *Finally, in the end, everything kind of came to a head. . . . I had been working hard, and one night I came home late. The house was dark and the kids were asleep already. I picked up the telephone and I heard a conversation between Jason and some woman . . . obviously something was going on. It was one of those conversations where you pick up and you hear a couple of seconds and you know exactly what's going on. He didn't hear me pick up the telephone. I went upstairs and he jumped straight up in the air when he saw*

me and I'm thinking, "Ummm, this is not right." First when I hear it, it's not right. Then I come in here and his reaction to seeing me isn't right. So, I confronted him then. I said, "Is something going on between you and this woman?" And he said, "No, no, no, no." He's laughing and "No, no. Nothing's going on." But you know in your heart something's going on. So, everything was just kind of, you know, falling apart. . . . Jason betrayed me in every way he could as frequently as he could.

Celeste's marriage disintegrated at the same time that she was having trouble at work. The combined stress of being betrayed by her husband—whose behavior she had tolerated for years because that was what she thought she was supposed to do—and of being let down by a job that wasn't all she was told it would be, triggered the most severe depression Celeste had ever experienced. Depression and low self-esteem made Celeste blame only herself for her current situation. Though she knew, intellectually, that her husband's behavior was inexcusable, she blamed her problems on her tendency to make bad choices. She made a plan to commit suicide by overdosing on prescription antidepressants. She was hospitalized as a result.

I thought it was probably my fault some kind of way. I felt that I must be provoking somehow . . . I needed to be more understanding . . .

I couldn't deal with the fact that a lot of my life choices were bad. First my marriage . . . then a job that I was working extra hard in and it wasn't satisfying and there wasn't any respect in it. It's like I was getting nothing.

I didn't believe in divorce. I hate to say this because back then, I wouldn't have admitted consciously that I felt this way. But now, looking back, I realize that I kind of looked at people who divorced as if they didn't try long enough. I always believed that if you tried hard enough you could make things work. So, divorce really wasn't an option. To me, when I got married, I got married for life. And I was just hoping and praying that if I kept working at it, that it was going to work out.

Celeste and Jason's relationship certainly drove her self-esteem to a new low, but Celeste had low self-esteem before she met Jason. Her high school experiences also made her feel lesser-than, but is this where her problems with self-esteem started? Probably not. They seem to have started much earlier.

My mother is very demanding in her way, especially with me. She had very high expectations of me. And it was hard on me. My mother gave [my siblings] more emotional support . . . I got more demands. She kind of put that image in me that I was the self-sufficient one. I didn't need much emotionally, so I wasn't given much emotionally.

From this early, primary relationship, Celeste learned an important lesson that she carried with her into adulthood: No one, not even her mother, was going to take care of her emotionally. Other people's emotional needs always came first. She learned not to expect emotional support at a very early age. It is likely that, as a child, Celeste did not understand why her mother was more supportive of her siblings. As a little girl, she could only believe that she didn't deserve her mother's tenderness. As an adult, she didn't deserve anyone else's, either.

Keisha: Earning Love

Keisha's early childhood experiences also contributed to her low self-esteem. The youngest child in her family, Keisha had always felt inferior to her sister, Dawn. Dawn never did anything overtly to make Keisha feel this way. She was simply a hardworking, very bright girl who excelled in practically everything she tried. But Keisha felt as if everyone compared the two sisters—and Dawn always came out ahead. Keisha's teachers, who had taught Dawn years before, often went on and on about her sister's accomplishments. Keisha also felt that her parents never let her be self-sufficient. In therapy after her first serious depressive episode, Keisha started to explore some of her family's dynamics.

> I had this long bout of jealousy with my sister. . . . My brother was very demeaning toward me and very condescending and very . . . he was putting me down all the time and that affected me. [The therapist and I] talked about that, my role with my parents, how they treated me—like a baby. They didn't foster my independence.

Keisha's brother, Mark, also physically abused her. This affected how she felt about herself as well.

> Mark did a lot of really cruel things to me. He tried to suffocate me once. He locked me in a closet once. He really beat up on me. I was afraid of my brother and I would do anything to please him. I think that had a big effect on how I reacted to guys later on in my life.

When Keisha started dating, she found herself desperately wanting to please her boyfriends, just as she had wanted to please her parents, her teachers, and her brother. Breakups often sent her reeling.

> One boyfriend broke up with me before Christmas break. I was devastated. I really had my mind on getting back together. So, we came back [from break], I tried to talk it over and he was like no, no. Then that started it [the depression]. I was crying every day; I just didn't know how to handle it. I was really distraught, in despair, I was really anxious most of the time. I started losing weight—in total I lost about

eighteen pounds. I wasn't eating. I had friends who were helping me through it, but it was just so hard. One of my friend's father was dying of cancer, so I had to help her. I just felt like I had no resources to draw on for help.

It didn't help when her boyfriends, like her brother, did particularly cruel things to her.

The guy that broke up with me after my sophomore year, we were still sort of seeing each other. I was feeling depressed. This one particular time he asked me to come over and we were intimate with each other. Then he kissed me on the forehead and said, "You have to get out before my girlfriend comes. I don't want you to be seen leaving my room." I was devastated. That really flung me into depression. I felt like I was in love with this guy.

I went home for the summer. I couldn't finish out the semester, so they sent my finals home. . . . I just started getting really self-conscious again and really introverted. I didn't want to go out with anyone. I thought of suicide every day.

Because Keisha felt that she was constantly compared to her sister, her early family experiences made her feel that she had to earn her family's love, even if that was not objectively true. Keisha's parents did love her unconditionally. But Keisha *perceived* that they trusted her siblings more, that they loved her sister more because of her accomplishments, and that they ignored the fact that her brother abused her. The objective facts are, in some ways, less important than what Keisha felt, and she felt as if she occupied a lesser position in her family. Her low self-esteem is one result of this feeling, and this lack of self-esteem fuels her depression.

Elaine: A Broken Fairy Tale

Elaine's self-esteem was high for much of her early life, but her adult experiences ravaged it over the years. After each blow, Elaine tried to recover, but a history of trusting and being betrayed left Elaine with very few emotional resources by the time she reached her sixties. Depression was the ultimate result.

Elaine's early life held some painful memories. Her parents had a volatile relationship that was not the stuff that dreams are made of. Elaine remembers her mother actually cutting her father's face with a razor during one of their arguments. She also recalls taking her younger brother and hiding under the bed to escape the fighting. This violent environment has left enduring scars. Elaine believes her fear of conflict and fighting that developed as a child has contributed to her tendency to avoid conflict as an adult, which has sometimes allowed her to be taken advantage of. But her aunt and uncle rescued Elaine from that chaos when she was ten years old. From that point on, Elaine was raised to expect only the best from life. The butcher shop her aunt and uncle owned was an integral part of the tight-knit Black community they lived in, and afforded them status and a decent living. Elaine went to Catholic schools, and she was homecoming queen and valedictorian of her senior class. Young men were always at her door. When she was granted a full scholarship at a women's college, she accepted, becoming one of only three Black women at the school. Even this was not a problem. Elaine remembers feeling welcomed at the school; only one nun was overtly prejudiced, and the students were friendly enough. When she graduated from college in 1949, Elaine felt that the world was at her feet. A few years later, she married, and a little more than two years after that, she had her first child.

Elaine had no reason to expect that her life would take the turns it did. When she learned of her husband's affair only a few years after their daughter was born, she was devastated.

I had always lived a fairy-tale life. I thought marriage was going to be like it says in the books. I thought I was doing what was expected of me. The meals were always ready, I did all the cleaning. . . . I did all those things that supposedly made a good wife.

I became pregnant with Gina after we had been married eighteen months.

Gene, my husband, was working two jobs at first—he had one job with the city and another with the post office. He finally quit the post office when his probation period with the city was up. He often had to work late and on weekends. They worked on these trailers, and there were no phones on the trailers, so he couldn't call me. But I didn't think anything about it.

He had been working late all week. One night when he got home late, I, for some reason, went down to the car. I don't know why I went down there. . . . I say God sent me down there. I just had a feeling. In the glove compartment were all these letters from this woman. It turns out he had been seeing this woman in the next state, driving out to see her. I couldn't understand it. I thought I was doing everything to make him happy. I never would have expected him to have an affair.

I went back to my aunt's. Of course, his mother was crying and carrying on and telling me this was the wrong thing to do. So eventually, we got back together. We bought a house, and things seemed to be going along pretty well.

Elaine started working as a teacher later that year. She tried to pretend that everything was fine, that the fairy tale was intact, but she knew something was still wrong with her marriage.

I talked to Gene and told him something was wrong, something was missing. I couldn't put my finger on it. He sloughed it off. We had friends in from out of town one weekend. Our friend Marva pulled me aside and said, "Elaine, did you know that Gene is jealous of Gina?" I was shocked. It had never occurred to me that a man would be jealous of his own child. But the more I thought about it, the more sense it made. Gene was jealous of the amount of time I spent with Gina.

Unhappy and confused, Elaine drifted away from Gene. She had met Nat, a teacher at the school where she worked, the previous year. They had certainly noticed each other, though they only said hello when they passed in the halls. Things changed with the new school year.

Then, in September, Nat and I started having lunch together. And one thing led to another . . . that's all I can say. I guess I was unhappy, and I really didn't realize what was going on. He was married, too.

Naturally, Elaine and Nat's affair caused a great deal of pain and confusion. Gene could not accept Elaine's infidelity, even though he had been unfaithful himself. Elaine and Gene divorced, and Elaine moved into her own apartment. She continued to see Nat, who had also divorced and moved into a place of his own. Elaine felt as if she didn't know herself anymore. Who was this person who cheated on her husband with a married man? Certainly not her.

Being Catholic, I never expected that I would end up divorced, or that I would have an affair. I never thought I would do anything like that. Things got really messy. Gene, his family, and Nat's wife tried to get us fired. They followed us. They wouldn't leave us alone.

I went away for a few weeks. The doctor told me that I had to get away from that situation or I would have a nervous breakdown.

Another shock awaited Elaine when she returned from her trip. She had left Gina with Gene's family, and now they wouldn't let Elaine take Gina back. A custody battle ensued, with Gene's family accusing Elaine of being unfit. One day, Gina told Elaine that her father's family would never speak to her again if she went to live with Elaine, and asked her mother to drop the custody fight. Elaine did, and Gina stayed with her grandmother until she graduated from high school.

Of all the shocks Elaine had experienced, this was by far the greatest. Elaine could not have imagined that her husband would cheat on her, that she would have an affair, and that she would lose her daughter. But that is exactly what happened. Devastated, Elaine tried to move on. She saw Gina as much as possible. She and Nat married and had a daughter, Nona, a year later. Elaine was thrilled to have another child. But things soon began to spin out of control again. When they married, Elaine did not know that Nat had a drinking problem. She soon learned, however, that he was an alcoholic.

Over the years, Elaine dealt quietly with Nat's drinking and various financial problems. No one really knew how bad things were for her. Not even her friends knew what was happening behind closed doors. Elaine truly loved Nat, but the drinking wore her down. He came close to dying at one point and was hospitalized several times. When Nat did finally give up drinking, Elaine thought, *Thank God. Now things will be OK.*

Things were OK for a few years. But the next big blow came when Elaine found out that Nat was seeing someone else. The nightmare was happening all over again. Elaine tried to get Nat to go to counseling, but he refused. Betrayed, angry, and humiliated, Elaine granted Nat a divorce.

As Elaine sees it now, nothing in her life turned out the way she thought it would. Elaine had expected that by this point in her life, she would be living like many of her friends are— growing old together, traveling, retiring to someplace warm and beautiful. Instead, she is a sixty-eight-year-old, twice-divorced woman who lives alone in an apartment. She had expected her life to be something entirely different.

> *Until I got married, everything had a way of progressing nicely. I thought that it was going to be a perfect life. There wouldn't be any ups and downs. My aunt and uncle sheltered me from a lot of problems. . . . I wanted three to four children. I wanted a home. I wanted a husband who liked to take me out and paid attention to me, who made me feel like I was important in his life. . . . I thought when Nat and I moved into our second house that this was it. We had made it. We would never have to move again. . . . When I looked up at age sixty-four and realized that I had nothing, I couldn't believe it.*

Though Elaine describes her early hopes as being a fairy tale, they reflect what most of us want from relationships: love, comfort, security, honesty, and fidelity. Elaine felt she had held up her end of the bargain with Gene, and when he betrayed her, her world—and her way of looking at life—no longer made any sense. She had failed at the most important things a woman could do: She couldn't keep her husbands happy, she had lost her child, and she was growing old alone. After a succession of failed relationships and circumstances she would never have imagined, Elaine's self-esteem was virtually nonexistent. It became very easy for her to blame herself for her problems.

There are thousands of Black women like Elaine, Celeste, and Keisha. We all want to find that relationship that makes us feel loved, desired, needed, and respected. These are natural longings. But if there is anything to be learned from Elaine, Celeste, and Keisha, it is this: Good loving begins with loving yourself. After twenty years of an unhappy marriage, Celeste has now taken this lesson to heart.

*I just want to be happy. It seems like that should be some-
thing easy to do, but it's not. Just to be happy. Part of being
happy will be loving myself better, treating myself better, putting myself first, so that I'm involved in positive relationships. There are certain things I want to do in my career. A
lot of it is very foggy because it is the first time in my life
that I've ever focused on myself. I've always been focused
elsewhere to the extreme. And so, it's interesting to even start
thinking now about what my goals are after this. I'm going
to start from scratch. I've got to figure out what it is that I
want, what I want to accomplish.*

Low self-esteem can lead us into a succession of unfulfilling
relationships. These relationships can trigger (or worsen) depression. For the depressed Black woman, getting out of unhealthy, unhappy relationships is often the first step toward
healing. Repairing your self-esteem is the first step toward finding the kind of relationship that will sustain you, not tear you
down. As Black women, we must affirm that we are beautiful,
lovable, and valuable in the face of much that denies these
facts. It is a challege, but one that must be met.

5
. . . .

Ain't Nobody's Business:
Family Secrets, Shame,
and Depression

Black folks are good at keeping secrets. Growing up, most of us were admonished, "Don't put your business in the street," no matter what might have been going on at home. Family business was family business: not even friends needed to know everything. The only safe ear was God's.

This ain't-nobody's-business attitude plays itself out in many ways that might, on the surface, seem counterproductive. For example, if you are depressed and feeling suicidal, refusing to see a therapist or psychiatrist because it will mean airing your family's dirty laundry might have disastrous consequences. But cultural beliefs and practices—such as keeping family business in the family—exist for a reason. This one, like so many others, evolved as a way to preserve the integrity of Black families. African-American families have always had to prove that they are not the breeding grounds for deviance the rest of society says they are. If you listen to the conventional wisdom, you will hear that Black families are matriarchal, physically abusive, incestuous, drug-addicted, work-averse, welfare-dependent dens of iniquity. If something bad was going on at home, you'd better not tell anyone: it would only prove the myth.

As a result, we have learned to deny that things like child abuse, domestic violence, and alcohol and drug addiction happen in our families. We tell ourselves that child sexual abuse is white people's mess. We are taught the value of family secrets: Keeping a terrible secret might cause you great pain, but it is the price you must pay to keep the family together in the face of so many forces determined to rip it apart.

Of course, we know that abuses of all kinds *do* happen in Black families, just as they happen in all other kinds of families. Most of us have at least one family story of an alcoholic aunt, a battering husband, a sexually abusive uncle. But a great number of us find it too painful to admit the effects of all this abuse. In our trademark manner, we try to be strong, to overcome, to forget. We keep our secrets. Abuse is rarely truly forgotten, however. It often remains buried in the subconscious, where, over time, memories of abuse evoke anger, rage, self-loathing, and depression.

No woman is strong enough to bear abuse and humiliation without ill effects—no human being is that strong. While we may valiantly try to go on with our lives as if nothing happened, abusive experiences change us. They may make it difficult for us to trust others, to develop healthy adult relationships, and to love ourselves. Women who were abused as children suffer many emotional and psychological difficulties, including anxiety and panic attacks, post-traumatic stress disorder (the disorder most often associated with Vietnam veterans), and chronic depression. Abuse survivors often self-medicate with alcohol and other drugs. They are twice as likely to be raped, sexually harassed, or battered as women who were not abused as children. Abusive experiences do not just go away because we don't talk about them. They fester. Talking about our secrets—bringing the violence, abuse, and addiction out in the open—is the only way to begin healing.

"I Brought You Into This World and I Can Take You Out": The Difference Between Positive Black Parenting and Child Abuse

With today's youth in ever-increasing jeopardy, we are beginning to hear more about getting back to the old ways of raising children. No more of this permissive Dr. Spock stuff, we say. Let's return to raising our children "the Black way." That'll make them mind.

But what do we mean by raising our children "the Black way"? Do we mean teaching them to respect themselves and their elders, to speak only when spoken to, to "honor thy father and thy mother"? These are positive parenting practices relied upon by generations of Black parents. Or do we mean returning to the days when Grandma sent you out to the yard to pick the switch she would beat you with? While switch whippings may have been the norm (or at least more acceptable) back in those days, we now recognize these often brutal beatings for what they are: child abuse.

Many of our parents were raised this way. They tell us, "By today's standards, I was an abused child," and they point out that they are just fine, thank you. And they are right. By today's standards, many of them were abused, and many of them quietly suffer. Some do not realize the ill effects this type of discipline had on them. Also, times were different then. While threats to Black children's self-esteem (and threats to their lives) were plentiful once they left the community, Black children were nurtured by the intact Black communities of our recent past. Segregation did have certain benefits, and one of them was that Black children were at the center of very vital communities where the "it takes a village to raise a child" principle was a guiding force. Even if there was trouble at home, most Black children felt loved and cared for by their extended families, neighbors, and communities. Extended family would often intervene when parents lost control or could not cope for some reason.

By contrast, children today are often the most victimized and least protected members of our communities. In neighborhoods where gangs, drugs, and drive-by shootings are commonplace, home is the only safe place for children. And when children live in fear of being abused by their parents, not even home is safe. A child who grows up without a sense of safety, of being loved and protected by those around her, grows up with fear and suspicion. She may find it hard to trust or get close to others, which can lead to loneliness and isolation in childhood and later in life.

Most tragically, children who are abused at home and who find no nurturing elsewhere believe they are unlovable. Abused children, like all children, try to make sense of their experience. While it might seem logical that they should be angry with or even hate the parents who abuse them, most never do. They spend their lives trying to understand why they were hurt by Mom or Dad. Young children, especially, have a psychological need to see their parents as perfect. Instead of placing the blame for the abuse on their parents, abused children believe that they somehow bring the abuse upon themselves. They become convinced that they are bad, evil, clumsy, or stupid. Abused children grow up believing the worst about themselves, and as a result usually have poor self-images and very low self-esteem, frequently persisting into adulthood. These early abusive experiences are the fertile ground in which depression takes root.

No Safe Place

Latrice

Latrice knows firsthand how abuse can all but destroy your self-esteem and sense of hope. Latrice grew up with a physically abusive, controlling mother, and was subjected to her mother's unpredictable violent outbursts throughout her childhood. She was also abused by her brother and was the victim of repeated sexual assault beginning at age five. Latrice is just now coming to terms with the effects of this abuse. Her story resonates with anyone who has survived childhood abuse.

> *My mother feels like "No matter how old you get, you'll always be a child and you have no right to tell me where I wronged you." It's real weird that I'll cuss out somebody on the street who wrongs me in a minute. But with my mother and my brother and anybody else who has wronged me in my family, I'll think, "I don't want to hurt their feelings."*
>
> *I never told my mother she was hurting me. I would just be quiet and hope that it would be over soon. I was never a teenager who talked back to my mother. When my mother said, "Be home at ten," I'd come home at ten and if I was late, then I'd just get my butt-whipping. I wouldn't be like, "Oh, Mom, let me explain." There was none of that for me.*

One particularly brutal beating occurred when Latrice was twelve years old. Her grandfather—who was in many ways mother and father to Latrice and her brother, Marcus—had suffered a stroke. Latrice was suddenly responsible for all sorts of things she had never learned to do because her grandfather had always taken care of them.

> *Up until that point, my grandfather did everything for me and my brother. He washed our clothes. I'd come home from school and my room would be completely cleaned, bed made, fresh linen or uniforms ironed, you know, everything . . . toys in the toy chest, dresser looking like a little girl's dresser. And my grandfather had dinner at least on its way to being done. He washed the dishes after dinner. So my brother and I did not learn how to do chores like most little kids coming up.*

But after my grandfather had the stroke, my mother came home one day and was like, "Wash the dishes." And I'm thinking, "Okay, I've seen Grandpa do this before. I think I've got it." So, I took this skillet, one of the cast iron skillets, and I washed the inside of it. I rinsed it off and I put it in the dish rack. My mother came over and touched it and she said, "It's not clean" and put it in the dishwater. I said, "Okay, well maybe I left something in there." And I washed the inside of the skillet again, rinsed it off. I'm thinking it's all clean, and I put it back in the dish rack. And my mother came and touched it again, and she's like, "This is not clean!" She did not tell me why it was not clean, where she was feeling dirt or anything like that. She just kept telling me to wash it again. So the third time, I washed it and I put it in the dish rack and my mother touched it and it was still dirty. The next thing I knew she had punched me in the nose and I started bleeding, all over the dishes, all in the sink. And my mother still did not tell me why that skillet was dirty. I did not know at twelve years old, having never done house chores, that you have to wash the outside of the skillet too in order for it to be clean. Seeing all of this blood, I freaked out. I had never had my nose busted before in my life. The blood was all in the sink, all on the dishes, all on my clothes, all over the floor. My mother just had this mean look on her face and said, "Make sure you clean up all that shit." I felt like she didn't care about me. I didn't think that she could sit there and bust my nose and not be like, "Oh, my God, I didn't mean to hit you that hard" or anything like that.

Latrice understands why her grandfather sometimes spanked her when she got out of line. But she detected something else in her mother's blows: rage.

There have been times that my grandfather just took off his belt and whipped me. But it was like, "Okay, well, yes I screwed up. I did wrong. I know I had no business doing it," and it was okay. But when my mother hit me, it was different.

When my mother would hit me or my brother, she would hit us like we were fighting and not like she was trying to discipline us. She used to ball up her fist and punch, and she would pick up whatever was around to hit you with. I just always felt physically abused. I always felt like this is not the way somebody should be hitting you.

Latrice's mother seemed to have a need to grind her daughter into the ground, to not only hurt her, but to humiliate her totally.

One time my mother beat me with a high-heel shoe for opening her mail. I realize that I was in the wrong and that I had no business opening her mail . . . but it was so humiliating because she was hitting me hard . . . she was hitting me so hard, I wet myself.

No one else knew how violent Latrice's mother could be, and Latrice never told anyone, not even her grandfather. She felt he had too many other, more important, things to worry about.

At the time that all of this stuff was going on, my grandmother was dying of Alzheimer's. And my grandpa had left his job and he was trying to take care of me and Marcus and my grandmother. He didn't need any more stress in his life. And besides, how was he going to deal with my mother? He couldn't chastise her about how she was raising her kids.

It was always going to be my word against hers or Marcus's word against hers. Everything was always so damn sneaky. My stepfather and my mother have been married for almost ten years. My stepfather has never heard my mother chastise us. He's never seen her hit us.

As she grew older and stronger, and as her anger toward her mother intensified, Latrice found it difficult to allow her mother to beat her. Bigger and stronger than her mother, it was only a matter of time before Latrice lost control.

Once I got into my teens and I started to realize that my mother could not fight, I decided I wanted to be adventurous. But I never had the heart to be mean to her, to take things to the extreme like she did. One time I was going to jump on her. I had been suspended from school, and my mother had grounded me. But my grandfather sent me to the bank for him. I came back, and my mother had beaten me home. And she says, "So, where were you?" I said, "Excuse me?" She said, "Why weren't you here when I got home?" And I said, "Because Grandpa sent me to the bank." I felt like, you know, that's easy enough. And she goes, "Well, what did I tell you to do?" "You told me that I was grounded." And she's like, "So, where were you?" "Grandpa sent me to the bank." And then she goes, "Well what did I tell you to do?" I got confused because I thought, "If my grandfather is here and he's the person I should be listening to, then if he says get up and go to the bank, then that's what I should do."

At that point, I was not paying attention to her because it got redundant. She got pissed off and she went to snatch the magazine out of my hand. She snatched it in a way that I got a paper cut across the face. Then she hit me in the face with the magazine. And at that moment, I lost all control. When she hit me in the face with the magazine, it was like, "That's it. I'm sick of this. I'm gonna jump on her." It just so happened my grandfather heard me jump up, but he thought somebody was falling or something. He came up and he saw me, and I think I might have had my mother's shirt in my hand and I had my fist drawn. And my grandfather was like, "Latrice, don't hit your mother. Don't hit your mother." I could see the fear in my mother's eyes. And I wanted so bad just to mess her up. Because I felt like, you know, you messed me up.

Latrice recognizes the intergenerational cycle of abuse in her family, noting that her grandmother lashed out at her in much the same way her mother did. (It is very likely that Latrice's mother was also abused as a child.) Latrice knows that her mother has let up on the beatings because she is afraid that Latrice might retaliate, but wonders if her mother will try to harm yet another generation, should she have the opportunity.

I was sitting in the high chair. You know how little kids mess over food and they're like, "Okay, I'm finished." Well, all of the women in my family are like clean your plate or you can't get up from the table. I remember sitting there telling my grandmother that I did not want to finish my cereal, I was full. And I remember her knocking me and this chair over because I would not finish these Frosted Flakes.

Sometimes I get to a point that I think when I start having kids, I don't want my kids around my mother because I don't want to put them in that kind of danger. . . . I don't think God would want me to feel that way, but I wouldn't put my child in that type of danger, either. So, I'll let my children visit my mother, but only if I'm there.

From their mother, Latrice and her brother Marcus learned that violence is an acceptable way to resolve conflict. Latrice and Marcus have always had a stormy relationship. Their cons-

tant fighting has contributed to Latrice's feeling that "someone is always doing me wrong."

*Marcus and I used to fight all the time. I wanted to fight
him back, but I always thought that I would hurt him. So,
I wouldn't fight him hard. Meanwhile, Marcus would do
all kinds of stuff to me. One time he lit a pack of firecrackers
and ran in my room and jumped in the bed with me. The
firecrackers went off, and I had burns all over my face, neck,
and chest. We used to beat each other with broomsticks and
mop handles. I would want to knock his head off. But I'd
just get this feeling like, "Man, if you hit him too hard and
hurt him . . ." It's like it never occurred to me that he was
beating the shit out of me just as hard as I wanted to beat
the shit out of him. I would just tell him, "Okay, stop."*

*One time I had some Vaseline on my face and Marcus
unscrewed a lightbulb and put it on my neck. There was
some electricity in the bottom of the light bulb and I got a
charge all through my face from him doing that. And it was
something that he thought was funny. He would take pliers,
hold a nickel or a quarter over the fire and then throw it to
me. I didn't see that it was coming off a fire and my first
reaction was to catch it. Or he would just drop it in my
hand or drop it on my hand or something like that.*

*Once he smothered me with a pillow. That was scary be-
cause I'm asthmatic. You have the sensation of being smothered with a pillow and then to have somebody actually
smother you with a pillow—it was terrifying. And Marcus
would say, "You're just taking it too hard" and "You're too
sensitive."*

*I could never injure Marcus the way that Marcus has
injured me. I don't know why I always protected him. Sometimes I think it's because I thought I would get into trouble
for hurting him. I just never wanted to hurt him.*

Maybe I was just scared that if I hurt him real bad that

he would hurt me worse. Now, when Marcus does stuff that I don't particularly care for, I have a mouth and I can say what's on my mind. But it's like, "Man, if I tell Marcus, I'm going to really hurt his feelings." So, I won't say whatever it is to him.

I don't think that Marcus did these things to be malicious. Now, I could be wrong. But it was always something that he thought was funny that really was abusive, you know. When Marcus and I would have these fights, my mother would just say, "Well, they're just killing each other."

In addition to being physically and emotionally abused by her mother and tormented by her brother, Latrice was sexually abused throughout her childhood. The abuse began when she was only five years old, when Latrice was sexually assaulted by her baby-sitter's cousin.

It seemed like every time I was at the sitter's, he [the abuser] was there. But he didn't live there. He had a party where he invited some guys from the neighborhood and they raped me. And from that instance on, it was like if all of a sudden you want to have sex with a child, there's the girl. I was being attacked at all kinds of places. Like going up through the hallway and getting attacked, trying to get home. Going up to my friend's house and getting attacked. Being at a friend's house and getting attacked. It became so common that I started thinking, "Well, I guess this is what I'm supposed to be doing." I was more used to being raped and being molested than not because it was happening so often. It went on until I was nine, when we moved to a different neighborhood. I thought, "Thank you, Jesus. I can't believe we're finally leaving." I stopped getting raped when we moved, and it was a big sigh of relief. Because it was something I had lived with. It was not something I was comfortable with.

But it was something I accepted. And for some reason, I knew moving was going to stop it.

Confronted with such overwhelmingly horrible abuse, Latrice could only imagine that it was somehow normal. Her mind could not allow her to see that she was being victimized repeatedly at such an early age, and that no one could protect her. It was too much for a child to bear. So Latrice, like many (if not most) women who were sexually abused as children, buried the abuse. She did not begin to acknowledge it until she was much older.

Memories of the abuse began to resurface when Latrice started having sex.

I put it out of my mind. I was in my teen years and I never thought about it. It wasn't something that I dealt with until I started having sex with my fiancé and then all of a sudden I could envision it. I'd get sick to my stomach. I was trying to tell my fiancé, "It's not you. I don't know what it is. But I can't have sex with you."

Her boyfriend's supportive reaction seemed to enable Latrice to explore the memories she had buried for so long.

He was cool about it. "Well, if I never have sex with you again, I'll always love you." It's not the reaction that I expected from a guy, but it was something that I guess I really needed to hear. It was like, okay, now I started to remember what was going on and the things that had happened to me.

I started telling people. I told Marcus when I was twenty. I still haven't told my mother. I told my grandfather. Everybody I tell is shocked. I'm thinking, "Why didn't you know?" My brother wanted to tell my mother, and I'm like, "No, she should know, she should know." But I don't think she does. She knows of one incident where I got gang raped in the

library because the librarian called. But I was telling Mar-
cus, now that I think about it, I got gang raped in the library
and I don't remember going to the hospital for it. I don't
remember being seen by anybody regarding the issue. It was
something that got swept under the carpet and I just dealt
with it.

Latrice learned very early on one of the primary lessons of
life as a Black woman: Bad things will happen to you, and no
one will come springing to your aid. You will have to learn to
just deal with it. So she did what many Black female victims of
childhood abuse try to do—she put it out of her mind, or so
she thought. Of course, the abuse did not go away. It has left
a lasting impression that things were not the way they were
supposed to be, that something was terribly wrong and no one
knew how—or felt a need to—fix it.

Despite the fact that Latrice tried to deal with everything
that happened to her, she could not. She remembers feeling
depressed quite often as a child, and she had no one to talk
to about how she was feeling or why.

I just felt sad, you know . . . Things would happen and I
really didn't know how to deal with them, but I'd just sit
there and think about them and let them eat away at me.

Then, as now, Latrice retreated into her room—and into
herself—when she became depressed. Food was a source of
solace, as it is for numerous Black women in emotional distress.
Her weight gain may have been a kind of armor, a way to keep
others from getting too close to her.

I was always overweight as a kid and I was always at home
by myself, or in my room by myself. My room was my sanc-
tuary. Even now, whenever I'm feeling sad, I stay in my
room. I don't deal with anybody. When I was a kid, I used

to always do that. I would sit in my room and read a book or sleep—mostly sleep.

Latrice is most certainly a strong woman. In many ways, it is amazing that she has survived. But she has not come through this trial by fire unscathed. She will live with the effects of the abuse she suffered for the rest of her life. Her depression is a logical response to being denied that which is every child's birthright: A safe and happy childhood, filled with love, trust, and growth.

Maya

Maya, too, has lived through abuse that has undermined her self-esteem and her ability to trust. While the abuse was not as long-lasting or pervasive as that Latrice suffered, the effects were just as serious.

We lived in my aunt's building. My aunt sexually abused me until I was about eleven. It would happen sporadically and I never knew when it was coming.

My aunt was an extremely abusive person. If I was in the bathroom and I had the nerve to lock the door, she would start banging on the door, saying, "This is my house, why do you have to lock my door?" That's when I got this sharp tongue because I learned how to say, "Because I'm using the bathroom in your house and I have locked your door and I am not unlocking it until I am through."

She would do things just to intimidate me. If I was in the tub and I had forgotten to lock the door, she would come in and pretend to like she was washing her hands or something and she would stand there for a long time while I was in the tub because she knew that I was body shy—just to intimidate me, just as an abuse.

Maya did tell her mother about the abuse, but her mother was an alcoholic, and either could not or would not truly grasp what was happening to her daughter.

> *I didn't know how to tell my mother that her sister had been touching me. I would say stuff to her and I could not articulate it exactly. I'd say things like "It makes my skin crawl and you know I hate it. Can't you get her to stop touching me." But my mother was not all there at that point, and she would say, "Well if you are having a bath, then she has to touch you." I'd tell her, "No she doesn't, I'm big enough to wash myself."*

Because of her alcoholism, Maya's mother never did anything to stop the abuse, leaving Maya to fend for herself. Her strongest response came years later, when Maya told her mother that this same aunt was abusing her own granddaughter. Though Maya was encouraged that her mother felt the need to say something, she couldn't help but wonder why her mother didn't stand up for her when she was being abused.

> *I would tell my mother things like this but she never took it seriously until I got to be older. When was eighteen or nineteen years old, I told her, "I hate your sister. I think she is a monster and I've seen her playing with my little cousin, touching her where she shouldn't be touching her." Well I guess she started taking me seriously then because she backed me up.*

The fact that Maya's mother did not come to her aid or protect her when she was being abused left Maya feeling alone and betrayed. Like Latrice, she turned to food for both comfort and protection.

I started gaining weight and getting bigger. The weight is what kept my aunt from physically abusing me anymore because I started pushing back.

In addition to touching her, Maya's aunt projected her own feelings about sex onto Maya. Instead of accepting responsibility for what she was doing to her niece, she tried to make Maya believe she was responsible for the abuse by belittling her and trying to make her feel dirty and ashamed.

If I asked any question at all about sex, my aunt had to say something about it. I would ask things like "where do babies come from?" Normal eight-year-old questions. My aunt would look at me as if to say, "See, I told you she is filthy. My kids wouldn't even think of asking anything like that until they were thirteen or fourteen years old. Why is she asking this at eight years old? Why does she need to know this?" When I got to be eleven and I came on my period, I wanted to use tampons. Apparently my mother mentioned it to my aunt or something—this was when my mother was drinking so if I told my mother she automatically told her sister. She said, "Well, you haven't been with any men, have you? What do you want to use tampons for?" I didn't understand. What does being with a man have to do with using tampons? I had been reading all the literature with the little preteen packages that Kotex would send you. I was getting all the information from that and I didn't relate it to anything about being with men. When I was fourteen, I remember wanting to go Christmas shopping with my friends. My mother said that I could go. It was after school and it was wintertime and of course it was going to be dark. My aunt immediately said, "It will be your fault if she gets pregnant." I said, "I don't understand. I'm going Christmas shopping with my girlfriends. How can I get pregnant going Christmas shopping with my girlfriends?" She associated everything with sex. Everything with her had to relate to sex and how filthy she thought sex was.

Victims of abuse, especially sexual abuse, frequently feel dirty and ashamed. Some carry these feelings—and the depression that results—with them their entire lives.

Latrice and Maya are just two of the countless women who have survived childhood physical and sexual abuse. We can no longer let these horrors be secret. We must begin to speak about our experiences of abuse, for ourselves and future generations of abuse survivors. We must acknowledge the things we have endured and what they have done to us—how abuse has left many of us bereft of hope, unable to trust or to connect to others, addicted, ashamed, depressed, and suicidal. Only by talking with someone about the abuse can we begin to make the connections between abuse, depression, and self-destructive behavior.

We must also recognize that some experiences are too painful and difficult to manage alone, and they require professional help. The kinds of horrors endured by abuse survivors are such experiences. We strongly believe that most, if not all, abuse survivors need help from a qualified mental health professional in order to heal. Many women think they can cope with this pain on their own, but for most it is simply too hard. There is no shame in admitting that you have been victimized and that you need help. Asking for help when you need it is actually a sign of great insight and strength. If you have been physically or sexually abused, if you are currently being abused, or if you do not remember being abused but suspect you might have been, therapy can help. See chapter 8 for advice on how to find a therapist who can help. We must make it safe for Black women to call abuse by its rightful name, to name our abusers, and to get help for ourselves. Keeping silent must no longer be an option.

6

· · · · · · ·

Lay My Burden Down:
Black Women and Suicide

I should like to die in winter
When my blood upon the snow
Will leave a clue to those who pass
Of my brief, futile life.

The garnet stain like a Rorschaht [sic] test
Will lead each to his conclusion.
"Too much, too soon" one will say.
"Too little, too late," will say another.

And none will learn the truth of the matter.
My secret will melt with the snow.
But the spot will run red each winter hence.
Though I be rotted below.

These sorrowful, bleak (and prophetic) words were written by the late Leanita McClain when she was just a teen-ager. The youngest columnist and editorial board member of the prestigious *Chicago Tribune*, the first African American and only the second woman to hold such a powerful position at the paper, Leanita McClain was one of journalism's brightest rising stars. But the depression that is evident in this poem eventually caught up with her. Almost twenty years later, at age thirty-two, convinced that her life was indeed futile, Leanita McClain took an overdose of antidepressants and died. She had just been named one of *Glamour* magazine's Women of the Year for 1984.

Thirty years earlier, another bright star, actress Dorothy Dandridge, was the center of attention in Hollywood. The tremendously gifted and stunningly beautiful Dandridge had just become the first Black woman to be nominated for an Academy Award, for her performance in the Black musical *Carmen Jones.* But neither Hollywood nor the rest of America was ready for a true Black leading lady. Three years would pass before Dandridge would be offered another leading role, and the roles she was offered were the ones America could deal with: the sultry Black temptress, the Jezebel. Even her role in *Porgy and Bess* was beneath her dignity. Despite the fact that *Newsweek* magazine had praised her as "one of the outstanding dramatic actresses of the screen," Dandridge only acted in two more films after *Porgy and Bess.* After two failed marriages and a bankruptcy, her personal life held little happiness for her, either. In 1965, at the age of forty-three, Dorothy Dandridge took an overdose of the antidepressant Tofranil, and died.

Writer Terri Jewell also seemed to be a success. At forty-one, she had just published her first book, a collection of quotations by Black women called *The Black Woman's Gumbo Ya-Ya.* She was also working on two more books. She was busy as one of the founders of Yahimba, an organization of Black lesbians, and was active in many social and political causes. Maybe Terri Jewell stayed so active to keep her depression at bay. A sexual abuse survivor, Jewell had persistent severe depressions, especially around the holidays. She would often check herself into the hospital when she felt the depression taking hold. But in 1995, Terri Jewell got tired of fighting. She went to one of her favorite parks, wrote her last journal entry, and shot herself in the head.

One of the last true R & B divas, Phyllis Hyman, will live forever in songs like "You Just Don't Know (What I've Been

Going Through)." Her music is all we have of her now. Also chronically depressed, Hyman had been struggling a lot in the last few years. Though she had a new album coming out, she had spent the last year recuperating from a foot injury that had kept her from performing in a musical. Her long-rumored problems with alcohol worsened, and she had gained a great deal of weight. All this combined to make Hyman feel lonely and hopeless, feelings she was already too familiar with. Just a few days before her forty-sixth birthday, Phyllis Hyman wrote a note, telling the world that she was tired. She then took an overdose of sleeping pills and never woke up again.

Myth has it that Black women do not kill themselves. We like to believe that things never get that bad, that none of us is ever that alone, that desperate. We hold on to one tragically misleading belief: *We are stronger than that.* The myth again keeps us from acknowledging the truth: We cannot bear everything, all the time. We do break down. Black feminist scholar and writer bell hooks writes about this myth in her book *Sisters of the Yam: Black Women and Self-Recovery.* "For years, many Black people perpetuated and believed the myth that Black folks did not commit suicide. That is a myth that is now brutally shattered by the overwhelming evidence that Black folks—women, men and children—are killing ourselves daily. Still, in a context where suicide is still seen as a sign of weakness, a character flaw, it is difficult for individuals to 'confess' suicidal states and suicidal feelings."

As hooks points out, we are killing ourselves daily, in both obvious and not-so-obvious ways. Black women actually have a lower completed suicide rate than other demographic groups (white women commit suicide at three times the rate of Black women; the rate for Black men is eight times as high, and for white men it is fourteen times as high). But these statistics do not include suicide *attempts*. The number of Black women who *try* to kill themselves is probably much higher than the number who actually succeed (this is even more likely considering that women have higher suicide attempt rates than men, but men have higher suicide completion rates). And for every Black woman who takes her life in a moment of despair, there are probably hundreds who are killing themselves slowly with drugs, alcohol, and overeating. Add to that the numbers of us who are killing ourselves with malignant neglect—ignoring those chest pains, that lump in the breast, that cigarette-induced hack—and we have a true crisis.

Why do Black women kill themselves? The majority of Black women who commit suicide are probably severely depressed. Like McClain, they have fought the illness for most of their lives. They simply get tired of fighting. Some have never received treatment for depression. Others do not respond to one type of treatment, and never have a chance to try another. Ironically, many of those who kill themselves are beginning to get better: the depression starts to lift, and the depressed woman has just enough energy to devise and follow through on a suicide plan.

Many of the Black women who kill themselves seem to have everything going for them. Leanita McClain, Phyllis Hyman, Terri Jewell, Dorothy Dandridge—all were extraordinarily talented, professionally successful women who took their lives despite all their successes. The stress and pressure of being an intelligent and successful Black woman in a society in which *intelligent, successful Black woman* is considered an oxymoron, combined with a vulnerability to depression, helped end these lives too soon.

Many Black women who kill themselves have lived through so much pain that they cannot imagine a time when things will be better. Women who were repeatedly physically or sexually abused as children may see suicide as the only way to stop reliving the trauma of their childhood. Women who are victims of domestic violence are frequently robbed of their will to live by their batterers. They may reach a point where death seems to be the only way they will ever escape the violence of their daily lives.

Severe depression also makes things seem worse than they really are. Negative thoughts overwhelm any slight sense of hope the depressed woman may have. The glass is always half empty. According to some reports, Phyllis Hyman never could understand why people wanted to hear her sing. She never appreciated her own talent. Hyman could only see herself through her own dark lens. From her point of view, there were far better singers than she. They deserved the attention. Fans, reviews, the love of friends and partners—nothing could change Phyllis Hyman's perspective on Phyllis Hyman.

Such negative thought patterns are a classic—and dangerous—symptom of depression. These thoughts often run counter to objective reality, but the depressed woman is convinced that her negative view of her self, her life, and her world *is* reality. The risk of suicide grows as these thoughts become more entrenched: If all is bleak, what is the point of living?

Elaine speaks eloquently about the thoughts that led her to attempt suicide. It is hard to tell which came first: Did Elaine's depression make her feel as if the stresses of her life had become too much to bear, or did the cumulative stresses of her life bring about her depression? Whatever the case, by the time Elaine became depressed and retired abruptly, her thoughts had become her worst enemy. She came to the conclusion that only death would bring her peace.

> *When I got home and started thinking about what I had done, it really started worrying me. I thought, "I have all these bills. I can't pay these bills. Why did I do this?" So, I'm sitting there one day and I become more and more depressed, so depressed that I decide to go talk to my priest. I told him I felt suicidal, and he took me to the hospital.*
>
> *They gave me some medication and released me from the*

hospital after a couple of days, and I went back home. A week later, I took an overdose of the medication I was on. Then I decided I didn't want to die. My brother-in-law's son was at home. He took me to the hospital and they pumped my stomach there. I was sent to another hospital and I was there for seven or eight days.

I went home again. Then I began to think, think, think. "Here I am, sixty-five years old. I don't have anything. I don't have a home, I've worked all these years . . ." It just disturbed me to no end, that here I have worked all these years and this is what I end up with. Nothing. Not a place to live, nobody to care for me.

I had $4,000. I was going to leave that to my daughters. I left a note. I drove to the woods, and I took the medication I was on and a bottle of scotch. I went into this area where no one would find me, and I took all these pills and this scotch. After a while, I could see all these bright lights and I was going through this tunnel, just like they say in all those stories about near-death experiences, and then all of a sudden I just started vomiting. I walked over to this clearing where these people were having a picnic. I said, "Oh, I'm so sick. I just tried to kill myself. Would you get me to a hospital?" The men laughed. They said, "Oh, she's drunk. Leave her alone." And this one lady said, "No, she's not drunk," and she walked with me. Then one of her sons drove me to the hospital.

A year later, when Elaine had a fourth depressive episode, she was again tormented by negative thoughts. It was as if she suddenly could see the world only through dark glasses. Even her memories were filtered through them—as she saw it, there was no light in her life, and there never had been.

I started thinking again, thinking about what had happened to my life, that this was not the kind of life that I had planned for myself. I have a problem, I guess, with my friends. I've always said that I have lived a lie. On the outside, everybody would think that I was doing as well as they were doing, that my life was as calm as theirs, and yet there was all this turmoil in my life. But I put on such a good front that no one would know what was going on. So I was just sitting there thinking about all these things that were happening to me, and why they were happening to me. I just couldn't believe it.

Elaine now recognizes how close she came to dying. "But for the grace of God," she says, "I wouldn't be here today." Looking at her now, it is hard to imagine that such a vibrant, alive woman has been so tormented, so desperate to die. She was lucky—maybe blessed—that she didn't.

We can only wonder what might have happened if someone had been able to connect with Dorothy Dandridge, Leanita McClain, Phyllis Hyman, or Terri Jewell before they grew so tired of fighting. Elaine's first depressive episode didn't occur until she was in her sixties; each of these women had been depressed since their teens or early twenties. Fighting for most of your adult life takes its toll. We can't stop everyone who wants to kill herself. But we have to try.

Suicide Warning Signs
and What to Do About Them

I should have known. These four words are heard far too often, probably every time someone commits suicide. When a loved one kills herself, the survivors live with the guilt. "Why didn't I do something?" they ask. "Why couldn't I tell?"

Most of us can't recognize the warning signs of suicide. If we did, perhaps some of our sisters would be saved. We need to pay attention to and talk about all those little things that seem odd to us. Talking about suicide will not make someone kill herself.

Some Black women will succeed in taking their own lives, and each one who does is a tragedy. We cannot stop them all. But by acknowledging that Black women are not immune to suicide, by knowing the warning signs, and by not being afraid to talk about suicide with our sisters who are in pain, we may prevent one more Black woman from ending her life too soon.

Though not all people who think about, attempt, or complete suicide are depressed, up to 60 percent are. It may be hard to know if someone is thinking about suicide. They are not likely to tell friends and loved ones, "I am planning to kill myself." Even so, there are outward signs that indicate that someone is considering suicide. If someone says things like "You would be better off if I weren't around," or "I'm such a burden to you," or "What's the use of going on?" you should take notice.

Certain actions should also raise your suspicion. A person who suddenly gives away her favorite clothes, books, CDs or other possessions may be contemplating suicide. Remember, too, that accidents aren't always accidents. Many car crashes, falls, and overdoses that are labeled accidents are actually failed suicide attempts. Abnormally heavy drinking or drug use may also be an indication that a person is feeling suicidal. A person who starts buying large amounts of alcohol or over-the-counter drugs (like aspirin, Tylenol, sleep aids, or cold medicine) may be plotting a suicide attempt. You should also be concerned if medications or alcohol start to disappear from around the house. (Of course, these things could also be an indication of a substance abuse problem, but either way, you should take notice.) Purchasing or borrowing a gun is another warning sign, especially if the person has never expressed a desire for a gun or has been afraid of or against guns in the past.

One of the most persistent—and often deadly—myths about suicide attempts is that they are merely cries for help. *Anyone who tries to kill herself should be taken very seriously.* Suicide attempts are not cries for help. Though they do indicate that the person in question needs help, people who attempt suicide see no other way to relieve their pain. They are not trying to get attention; they are trying to end their suffering.

If someone close to you says she is tired of living, asks "What's the point of going on?" or tells you she is planning to kill herself, *heed the warning.* Telling her how wonderful she is and reminding her of all those who love her is nice, but it will not stop a suicidal sister from carrying out her plan. Neither will quoting the Bible and telling her that suicide is a sin. Suicidal thinking is not subject to rational discussion. Trying to talk a suicidal sister out of taking her life is not enough. Don't leave her alone. If she is seeing a therapist, find the number and call him or her. If not, call her doctor. Take her to an emergency room and stay with her. Be ready to explain what is going on to the hospital staff. Not all doctors and nurses understand depression, so you may have to do some on-the-spot education. Take this book with you.

If you are feeling suicidal, it may be hard to imagine that things will ever be any better. *They will.* If you have recurrent thoughts of suicide, call your doctor, therapist, minister, or priest immediately. If you are afraid you are going to hurt yourself, try not to be alone. If your suicidal feelings become unbearable, go to the hospital. You *can* feel better.

Despite the pain, our lives are worth living.

PART III

· · · · · · · · · ·

TREATMENT, SELF-HELP, AND PREVENTION

7

. . . .

What Causes Depression?

A debate is raging about the causes of depression. Some—most often biopsychiatrists (medical doctors who study and treat the biological bases of mental disorders)—believe depression is a purely biological disorder, caused by deficiencies of certain chemicals in the brain, hormones, or mistimed body clocks. Others—usually psychologists and other psychotherapists—think biology may be one piece of the depression puzzle, but psychological factors play a large role. Still others feel that social, cultural, and political factors contribute to depression.

For now, at least, no one theory can explain everything, and it is likely that the future will only confirm what seems the logical conclusion today: that depressive disorders have biological, psychological, and social components, and that episodes can be triggered by any number of internal or external events. This chapter explores the current theories of depression and looks at them in light of Black women's experiences.

The Biological Perspective

The biological perspective views depression as a medical illness with a knowable physical cause. Research into the biological causes of depression has been compelling, and it is now gen-

erally accepted that major depression and the other mood disorders are at least partly biological in origin. How big a role
biology plays and what that role is, exactly are slowly unraveling
mysteries for researchers who study depression and physicians
and therapists who treat it.

The Chemical Connection
One clear indication that there is a biological component to
major depression is the effectiveness of antidepressant medications—drugs prescribed to treat the illness. Antidepressants
appear to correct imbalances of certain brain chemicals that
are lacking (or poorly regulated) in depressed people. These
chemicals, called *biogenic amines,* facilitate communication between nerve cells in the brain. Biogenic amines are one type
of *neurotransmitter,* a class of chemicals involved in transmitting
the electrical impulses that dictate pretty much everything you
do (from breathing to walking to thinking and feeling) from
one nerve cell to another throughout the body. Very simply
put, the electrical impulses (or messages) travel down the nerve
cells, stimulating the release of neurotransmitters, which then
carry the impulses to the next cell down the line.

The neurotransmitters thought to be most involved in depression are *norepinephrine, serotonin,* and *dopamine.* Each of
these has a different role to play in the regulation of mood.
Researchers have found evidence that too little of any of these
neurotransmitters can cause depressive symptoms; too much
seems to trigger mania. The success of one class of antidepressant drugs, the serotonin-specific reuptake inhibitors (SSRIs)
like Prozac, makes researchers think that serotonin may be the
major player in many cases of depression. Some also believe
that there are different types of major depression caused by
abnormal levels of different neurotransmitters. In other words,
a lack of serotonin may cause a different type of major depression, with different symptoms, than a lack of norepinephrine. This would help explain why, to take one example, some

depressed patients have trouble sleeping, but others sleep too much.

Despite the elaborate theories, no one is certain as to how neurotransmitters may be involved in depression or how anti-depressants work to regulate these brain chemicals. Researchers in the fields of neuroscience and biopsychiatry are furiously working to find answers to these questions and to develop new, more effective drugs to treat what may turn out to be several different types of neurotransmitter-related depression. At this point, what we do know is this: There is some connection between neurotransmitters and depression. Hopefully, we will soon know what that connection is.

Hormones, Mood, and Depression

There is strong evidence that hormones may also contribute to depression. Research in this area has focused on the role of the hormones involved in the regulation of appetite, sleep, and adaptation to stress (those secreted by the adrenal glands); the thyroid hormones, which control metabolism; and the female sex hormones estrogen and progesterone.

The thyroid gland. Thyroid gland malfunctions are one of the most common causes of depressive symptoms. For example, hypothyroidism (also called underactive thyroid) is caused when the thyroid gland produces too little of the hormone, and it can result in all the symptoms of major depression, including slowed thinking, fatigue, appetite changes, depressed mood, and suicidal thoughts. Most doctors will automatically test for thyroid hormone levels when a patient complains of these symptoms. If thyroid hormone levels are found to be low, hormone supplements will be prescribed (often in addition to an antidepressant).

The adrenal gland, cortisol, and the stress response. Psychiatrists have long noted that high levels of the adrenal hormone cortisol, which helps regulate sleep, appetite, and adaptation to stress, are found in the blood of depressed people. Some researchers think that these high cortisol levels reflect a malfunction in the body's stress-response system. Humans, like all other animals, have an internal alarm system that warns us when danger is near. When we are frightened or in danger, our bodies react with a stress response that is very similar to what happens in depression. For example, appetite and sexual interest decrease, the immune system is suppressed, and anxiety increases. (Though depression seems to slow thoughts and actions down, the mind is actually hyperaware during a depressive episode, obsessively focusing on feelings of inadequacy and guilt). This reaction, called the fight or flight syndrome, prepares the body for dangerous or stressful situations. Cortisol is a by-product of this reaction. Therefore, the abnormally high cortisol levels might indicate that the body is in this high-stress state more often than it should be. Instead of shutting off once the danger has passed, the body remains in a constant state of stress, and areas of the brain that control the emotions involved with stress (and depression) are overstimulated. These high cortisol levels may also damage or destroy brain cells that regulate the stress response. This theory complements psychosocial theories of depression that hold that people who are emotionally, physically, or sexually abused in childhood often become chronically depressed. Such people may be in a constant state of high stress because their childhood experiences conditioned them to always be ready for danger.

Female sex hormones. For years, doctors have told women that the mood swings, crying jags, irritability, and appetite and sleep changes they experienced each month were just in their heads. Fortunately, male doctors' condescension toward female patients has been exposed, and researchers have started to take women's hormone-related complaints seriously.

The fact that many women have depressive symptoms before their periods makes some researchers think that the changes in hormone levels that cause premenstrual syndrome (PMS) and premenstrual dysphoric disorder (PMDD) may also have something to do with major depression (and postpartum depression) and may explain why women have higher rates of depression than men. Some researchers have found gender-related differences in how neurotransmitters function, and in thyroid and adrenal gland functions. They speculate that sex hormones may be responsible for these differences. When estrogen levels decrease (for example, after childbirth), the flow of norepinephrine, serotonin, and dopamine also decrease. This may trigger depressive symptoms in susceptible women. Birth control pills, which contain the hormone progesterone, may also be a cause of depression in some women, though the number is thought to be small. The fact that depression rates in girls begin to rise at puberty (when estrogen and progesterone levels increase dramatically) also supports theories relating depression to female sex hormones.

You Feel What You Eat: Diet and Depression

Theories linking diet and depression are controversial, but they are also quite intriguing. Low blood sugar (hypoglycemia) causes the release of insulin, which can trigger depressive symptoms. Diabetes, a condition in which your body lacks sufficient insulin (very common among African Americans), can also produce the same effect. Caffeine and carbohydrates like table sugar seem to trigger depressive episodes in people who are sensitive to sugar and caffeine.

Vitamin deficiencies can also cause depression or depressive symptoms. Vitamins—especially the B vitamins—have a profound effect on the central nervous system. Vitamins B_1 and B_6 (thiamine and pyridoxine) are directly involved in the production or regulation of neurotransmitters, while deficiencies of vitamins B_3 and B_{12} (niacin and cobalamin) can cause symptoms of depression and related disorders, like anorexia. Folic acid deficiencies can also cause depression. Minerals like sodium, potassium, iodine, and calcium are also needed for the nervous system to function properly; any serious mineral deficiency can lead to depressive symptoms as well.

Sleep and the Body Clock

Disturbances in the sleep/wake cycle are commonly associated with depression. Depressed people often report symptoms of disturbed sleep, most often complaining of insomnia, though hypersomnia (sleeping too much) is reported as well. Studies of sleep patterns in depressed people have shown that the type and quality of sleep is different than that of nondepressed people.

In some depressed people there may be discrepancies between the time of going to sleep and the activity of their biological clocks. The chemicals needed to regulate their sleep cycles—the hormones melatonin and cortisol—are either released at the wrong times (for example, early in the evening instead of at their later bedtimes) or in greater amounts than needed. This may cause the insomnia or hypersomnia a depressed person experiences.

Seasonal depressions like seasonal affective disorder (SAD) may also be related to the release of melatonin. For instance, as winter approaches and sunrise comes later and later, melatonin suppression also happens later. If the body does not adjust to this, the sleep/wake cycle becomes out of sync and depression may occur.

Though all the biological theories of depression seem to have some validity (some more than others), none explains everything. Furthermore, there is a chicken-and-egg question: Do the biological changes trigger depression, or does some psychological or social event trigger changes in emotion, which then cause physiological changes to occur? Also, while many of the biological theories of depression are plausible and make a lot of sense, many of them are still just theories and really have not yet been sufficiently tested.

It's a Family Affair:
The Genetic Perspective

Many studies have confirmed that major depression and the other mood disorders do seem to run in families. Some studies have found that people with first-degree biological relatives (parents or siblings) who have major depression are 1.5 to 3 times more likely to be depressed than the general population. Those whose first-degree relatives have *any* type of mood disorder are about 3.5 times more likely to have either a unipolar or a bipolar disorder themselves. Dysthymia is also more common among people who have parents or siblings with major depression. There is even stronger evidence of a family connection with the bipolar disorders: first-degree biological relatives of people with bipolar I disorder have 4 to 24 percent higher rates of both bipolar I disorder and major depression.

Research studies called *twin studies* provide some of the best evidence of a genetic component in mood disorders. These studies compare the rates of mood disorders in identical and fraternal twins. Since identical twins have exactly the same genes, any truly hereditary illness or condition should be present in each twin. This bears out for the bipolar disorders: if one twin has bipolar I disorder, the chances that the other twin will have some mood disorder is near 10 percent, and the chance that the mood disorder will be a bipolar disorder is 80 percent. In these studies, fraternal twins, who do not have the same genes, have the same rates of mood disorders as any other siblings.

The connection for major depression, however, is not as clear. One study found that when one identical twin is depressed, the other twin will develop the disorder in 40 to 78 percent of the cases, while the rate for fraternal twins is the same as for nontwin siblings: 0 to 13 percent. This indicates a strong—though not complete—genetic basis for major depression. If depression were truly a hereditary illness, both identical twins would be depressed in 10 percent of the cases. Since this does not happen, other environmental and social factors—like stress, psychological makeup, life history, nutrition, and other physical illnesses—clearly play a role in the development of depression. Most researchers currently feel that certain people may have a genetic predisposition to mood disorders like depression, but environmental factors help determine whether or not they will actually become depressed.

Why We're Black and Blue:
A Bio-Psycho-Social-Political View
of Depression in Black Women

Since the beginning of this century, mental health professionals have recognized and struggled to understand the illness we call depression. The earliest theories about the illness developed from clinical observations of people who were depressed. Practitioners reasoned that the depressed person was reacting to a traumatic loss, real or imagined, or suffering from displaced anger turned onto the self.

Over the ensuing years, the theories about reasons people become depressed have grown increasingly sophisticated. Remarkably, these two themes of loss and displaced anger have resurfaced in many contemporary theories of depression. However, few, if any, of the existing psychological theories of depression have sought to specifically examine the causes of depression in Black women. This is not entirely surprising, since Black women have never been high on anyone's research priority list. As a result, no one really knows how many of us are depressed at any given time. No one knows whether we are more or less susceptible to depression than anyone else, or if we have different symptoms. No one knows if the causes of depression are different for Black women. Until recently, few people thought to ask. We simply weren't important enough.

To be sure, there are many discussions about the conditions that are associated with depression and African-Americans' vulnerability to depression. For complex sociological and economic reasons, these conditions are overrepresented among Blacks. We can also look to our experience and to common sense to explain some of the reasons for our depression. For example, we know that African Americans are at greater risk for developing a virtual laundry list of ailments and illnesses: everything from breast cancer to heart disease to asthma and diabetes strikes us more frequently than whites. Of the sixteen leading causes of death, the mortality rate for Black women surpasses that of white women in thirteen of those causes. Common sense tells us depression is probably no different. Research points to the connections between living in a racist society and these illnesses. Common sense tells us that living in a society that places little value on our Blackness or our femaleness must take its toll on our psyches as well as our bodies. Research asserts that poverty and loneliness lead to isolation and depression; common sense says we are more often poor and alone, isolated and depressed. Research concludes that people in psychological pain often self-medicate with whatever is available: sex, food, drugs. Common sense points out that we would not need the salves we so often choose—unhealthy relationships, food, cigarettes, alcohol, and drugs—if our minds and souls were not pained.

The American Psychological Association's National Task Force on Depression and Women found that though depression does have some biological basis, certain life circumstances and psychological events can bring on depressive episodes. Specifically, overwhelming stress—from work, relationships, or parenting—is a significant risk factor, as is victimization (childhood sexual abuse, rape, domestic violence), inadequate income, alcohol and drug abuse, and violence. These events are disproportionately represented in the lives of Black women. For instance:

- The majority of Black women—including those who are married and those with young children—work outside the home.
- Fifty-seven percent of Black women never marry or are separated or divorced.
- Forty-three percent of Black mothers are single parents.
- Fifty-two percent of Black women live below the poverty line; another 15 percent are considered working poor.
- Alcohol abuse contributes to twice as many deaths among Black women as among white women.
- One in every four Black women will be a victim of sexual assault by age eighteen.
- Twenty-two percent of Black women are victims of domestic violence.
- The homicide rate for Black women is four times higher than for white women.

Other points to consider:

Several studies have shown that married women have lower rates of depression than single women. The companionship of marriage seems to protect women from the loneliness and isolation that can trigger depressive episodes. Since Black women are more likely to be single, separated, or divorced, fewer of us experience this protective effect of marriage. Also, Black women have much longer life expectancies than Black men (seventy-four years on average for Black women, sixty-seven for Black men). This means that a great number of married Black women will spend many years as widows, who are at increased risk for depression.

Working Black women (and that means most of us) face all the stresses working white women do (balancing work and family, trying to break through glass ceilings, fending off sexual harassment, and earning less money than our male counter-parts). In addition, we must grapple with stresses that are unique to us, such as being passed over for promotions because of racial discrimination, being thought of as the affirmative-action hire and having our abilities questioned, and facing the wrath of Black men who feel we are taking their jobs. Professional success is certainly no guarantee of happiness: When Black women move from lower-paying to higher-paying jobs, the incidence of depression actually increases. This might be because career success often means being separated from our support systems. Meeting new people and keeping up with old friends can be hard when you work sixty hours a week. And if those old friends don't have the same types of jobs, empathy and understanding may be hard to come by. Career success is a double-edged sword for many Black women: Our success sometimes estranges us from our families and communities when we need them most.

While disproportionately large numbers of Black women are poor, even those who make good money are often besieged with financial worries. We all know sisters who appear to have it together but in actuality are one late paycheck away from financial peril. Many of us feel responsible for family and friends who aren't doing as well as we are. If a sibling needs rent money or a niece's tuition must be paid, we feel obligated to do what we can (which is often more than we should). Those of us in the sandwich generation—who are taking care of our children *and* our parents—are especially hard-pressed. Few of our parents are able to adequately prepare for old age, which often makes us their main source of support. And many of us have learned the hard way that keeping up with the Joneses has its price. Designer clothes, luxury cars, and being seen in all the right places has led many a sister to bankruptcy and subsequent depression.

Research points to clear connections between the corrosive effects of living in a racist society and many life-threatening illnesses that plague African Americans. Common sense tells us that living in a society that devalues both Blackness and womanhood must take its toll on our psyches as well. Yet, how do we understand this theoretically? The theories of loss and displaced anger are interesting, but they do not adequately address the common psychological experiences of most Black women.

In contrast to the theories that explain depression in terms of loss or anger turned inward are those that purport that depression is a behavioral disorder that is the consequence of learned behavior. Psychologist Martin Seligman pioneered the well-known *learned helplessness* theory of depression. He argued that depression results when people have no control over their environments and give up the expectation that they will ever gain control.

According to Seligman's theory, life experience teaches people that any efforts they make to effect changes in their life circumstances are futile; nothing they do matters. Consequently, people learn that they are helpless and powerless and become resigned to their fate. These are our perpetual victims. The most vulnerable are people who have suffered repeated trauma. This includes women who have been physically or sexually abused over long periods of time; chronically impoverished women; and women who have experienced chronic discrimination and oppression. These are women who look battered and defeated by life (and, indeed, often they have been literally battered and defeated). They appear to have thrown in the towel.

Seligman feels that depressions are at an all-time high. He attributes this epidemic to the conditions of contemporary society. Seligman believes that the importance our society attributes to individualism and personal development has led to what he calls "the culture of maximal selves." This increases our vulnerability to feeling personally responsible for all our circumstances and failures. Another consequence of the maximal-self culture is a feeling of isolation and estrangement, for ties with the community are weakened as individuals seek for themselves and there is less community support in times of stress and failure.

Seligman's maximal selves theory seems to echo what the Afrocentric theorists have argued for years. The Afrocentric theorists—most notably Molefe Kele Asante of Temple University in Philadelphia—believe that African Americans' psychological well-being is fostered by living in a society that values the collective interests of its members more than the interests of any one individual. Accordingly, the mental health needs of African Americans fare poorly in the United States because of, among other things, the American emphasis on individual achievement and success, often at the expense of the masses. The Afrocentric theorists feel that cultures such as African ones, which value spiritual awareness and cooperation over materialism and competition, community over individuality, and interdependence over independence are better settings for optimal psychological growth and development.

The cognitive theory of depression, pioneered by Aaron Beck, also emphasizes the role of learning and thinking in depression. Beck and his supporters argue that depression is a disorder of thinking. Disordered thinking or *cognitive activity* influences the way we think about our circumstances and situations. These thoughts greatly influence our perceptions, behaviors, and feelings. People develop habitual styles of thinking about events called *cognitive styles*. These cognitive styles are characterized by certain *automatic thoughts*, which seem to kick in like a recording whenever something triggers them. We are all aware of women who frequently say and seemingly live by the dictum "It's never gonna get any better, so why try," or "All men are dogs so I might as well keep him; he beats being alone." According to cognitive theory, these habitual styles become self-defeating attitudes that are more likely to occur during stressful periods. The woman's perceptions are driven by her cognitive style, and this makes her vulnerable to becoming depressed.

We certainly recognize the value of the learned helplessness and cognitive theories in helping people understand depression. But we also think that a person's emotions and feelings and the messages she gets about herself from the world at large play a central role in the development of depression. After all, depression is a mood disorder, and moods are all about feelings. This may seem like semantic quibbling—feeling versus thoughts—but there is an important difference. One may claim to have optimistic, positive thoughts most of the time and indeed, if you ask someone what she's thinking, she will tell you things that sound positive. However, we know that we may think one thing and feel another.

Psychodynamic theories focus on both feelings and the effect of the environment on psychological development. Pioneered by the work of Sigmund Freud and developed by hundreds of theorists who have found the views helpful, psychodynamic theory places great importance on the role of early life experiences in current life difficulties. Psychodynamic theorists believe that the unconscious (thoughts, feelings, and desires of which you are unaware) influences behavior, and that unless early life issues are resolved, current problems with roots in those issues will persist.

The dynamic theories of depression are varied and unduly complicated. Rather than attempt an overview of psychodynamic theories of depression, many of which are now thought to be obsolete, we will focus on an early paper that *we* feel was a precursor to Seligman's theory, and a contemporary theory that we believe offers a useful way of thinking about and understanding the psychological worlds of Black women.

In the early 1950s, Edward Bibring wrote a brief paper on depression in which he held that "depression is essentially a human way of reacting to frustration and misery, whenever the ego finds itself in a state of real or imaginary helplessness against overwhelming odds." He stressed that "depression can be defined as the emotional expression of a state of helplessness and powerlessness." Bibring felt that when the ego feels it is prohibited from living up to its aspirations, it (the ego, hence the person) feels depressed. He believed that people had common strivings, such as the wish to be deemed worthy, loved, and appreciated and not inferior or unworthy; the wish to be strong, superior, great, and secure as opposed to weak and insecure; the wish to be good and loving, rather than hateful, aggressive, and destructive. Depressive feelings developed as a result of recurring events that sent a clear message to the ego (person) that the person was not valuable and was not going to be allowed to fulfill basic dreams. Though the depression often went into remission, people were vulnerable to recurrent episodes whenever they confronted circumstances that made them feel powerless and devalued.

Also during the 1950s, one of Freud's followers departed from traditionally Freudian ways of thinking about people's psychological well-being and development. Heinz Kohut began looking closely at human psychological development in relationship to real things that happened in their environments. Kohut and his followers gradually grew to understand that human development occurs in the context of real-life experiences that cannot be disregarded. If we are to understand human behavior, then we must understand the environments from which people come and the psychological effects those environments have on people's views of themselves. Kohut and his colleagues developed a theory examining human development and illness called *self psychology*. Like other well-developed theories of human development and behavior, self psychological theory is complicated. For our purposes, we will greatly simplify the theory and discuss the parts we think enhance our understanding of depression in African-American women.

Self psychologists define the self as that psychological structure which makes its presence evident by providing one with a healthy sense of self-esteem or well-being. Thus, the world in which one lives is of extreme importance in facilitating a feeling of well-being. If a person is to thrive and develop the capacity to soothe and calm herself during periods of stress, she must get certain self-sustaining, growth-facilitating, approving responses from the world early in life and consistently throughout life. When these confirming, validating responses are absent, the self (hence the person) is vulnerable to a host of psychological illnesses, including depression. Thus, according to contemporary self psychologist Ernest Wolf, while one is born with "certain potentials that are his biological heritage, it is the interaction with the environment that will evoke some of these potentials and bring them into development, whereas others are left to atrophy." Similarly, one can reason that the same biological potentials may remain dormant if one has optimal life experiences. According to Wolf, "if a person is to feel well, to feel good about himself with a secure sense of self, enjoying good self-esteem and functioning smoothly and harmoniously without undue anxiety and depression, he must experience himself consciously or unconsciously as surrounded by the responsiveness of others."

Afrocentric theorists have long held that the cumulative effects of living in a society where racism and discrimination prevail contribute significantly to depression in African Americans. Furthermore, living in a world that lauds white standards of beauty, speech, dress, and expression as the only acceptable behaviors and desirable ways to look is extremely destructive to Black women.

If we remember Celeste, her experiences at boarding school were unbearably difficult. At a time in her life when she greatly needed support and understanding from her peers, she was ridiculed and ostracized primarily because of her race. The world at her school was hostile, and—though it was undoubtedly unintentional—the world at home that she turned to for understanding received her complaints with deaf ears. Celeste stated that her mother (a key person in the development of our selves) was so eager for her to have a chance at the good life that she was unable to respond with empathy when Celeste told her about the painfully miserable experiences she had at boarding school. Tragically, a time of life that should have been adventurous, fun, and enlightening was overwhelming and destructive.

In the book *Two Nations: Black and White, Separate, Hostile, and Unequal,* sociologist Andrew Hacker points out that like it or not, being Black in America requires that one relinquish certain aspirations and dreams and, as he puts it, "learn it is safest to make peace with reality: to acknowledge that the conditions of your time can undercut dreams of enduring romance and 'happily ever after.' . . . This is especially true if you are a black woman . . ." Others have written poignantly about the subtle but insidious indignation to which Black people—men and women—are subjected. Sadly, all Black people have experienced firsthand overt and covert slights that leave us with complex feelings of humiliation, anger, and despair.

As we think about the world and its response to Black people, we are confronted with the sad realization that many of the messages Black women receive about themselves—both from the larger society and our families—are overwhelmingly negative and discouraging. To be sure, things have greatly improved since the 1960s, when the only media representations of people of color were demeaning caricatures. Black girls see Black women on television in a variety of professions, and dolls of every hue are available at the local toy store. But Black women and girls frequently pick up on quiet, subtle messages of inadequacy, inferiority, and uselessness in their daily life experiences. Demeaning myths about Black women abound. While we may not be more biologically predisposed to depression than others, we are, by our race, more often than not predisposed to a dubious reception from a world that, in general, has little positive use for Black people. This is hardly the kind of confirming, validating response that contributes to the growth of a vital self or a healthy sense of self-esteem.

Psychologically, we certainly seem to be vulnerable to depression. However, until we get some hard-core data about the incidence of depression among Black women, we can't be sure how great the numbers are. Certainly, we know of women who persevere in spite of repeated blows from a callous world. Resiliency is an asset that many people have, and it seems to be abundant in African Americans. We are survivors, and we know better than anyone that being Black is not for the faint of heart! We also know that being strong, proud, and able to tough it out are often masks for profound feelings of sadness that we do not feel free to disclose. We must find a way to express ourselves and get the responses we need from the world for our health's sake. We must also free ourselves from the burden of being strong when we feel frail; being proud when we feel defeated and humiliated; and being quiet when we want to shout to the world that we hurt.

8

· · · · · · · ·

There Is a Balm in Gilead:
Finding Treatment for Depression

Depression is a thief: it steals your energy, appetite, and desire. Most devastatingly, it steals your hope, leaving you with the intolerable feeling that things will never look bright again; that your life will never return to normal.

This is the big lie of depression. There *is* hope. As we have said throughout this book, most depressions can be treated successfully. Close to 80 percent of those who are treated for depression get better. However, we have also pointed out that most depressed people—especially depressed Black women—do not receive treatment of any kind.

You might wonder, *Why should I seek treatment for depression?* Well, the answer is simple. Clinical depression is an illness, like heart disease, diabetes, or cancer. Would you refuse to go to the hospital if you had a heart attack? Would you refuse insulin if you would go into a diabetic coma without it? Would you refuse chemotherapy if you had life-threatening cancer? Probably not. You would get treatment for your physical illness.

Unfortunately, most of us think depression, a mental illness, is different. We believe we should bear up under the weight of emotional and psychological pain because we are rarely given permission to feel bad. Because depression is a mental illness, we think our minds should be able to overcome it. We think we shouldn't need treatment for depression; that we should be able to snap out of it. But you can't snap out of clinical depression, just like you can't snap out of heart disease, diabetes, or cancer.

The National Mental Health Association's survey of African Americans' attitudes about clinical depression found that denial, embarrassment, and fear keep us from getting the treatment we need. According to the survey:

- **Forty percent of African-American respondents said they would not seek treatment because of denial.**
  African Americans have trouble admitting that depression can happen to us. We tell ourselves we are just tired, overworked, or stressed-out when we are actually depressed. "Black people don't have time to be depressed," we say.
- **Thirty-eight percent wouldn't seek treatment because of embarrassment or shame.**
  Many of us still equate depression with weakness, craziness, or a lack of faith in God. Admitting depression, we think, means admitting that you are unable to measure up, or, worse yet, that your belief in the Almighty has wavered. Bringing the shame of mental illness on our families is also a concern.
- **Thirty-one percent wouldn't want or would refuse help.**
  Those of us who refuse help for depression usually think we can overcome it ourselves. Others may not trust health professionals—perhaps for good reason—or may not believe that depression is an illness that can be treated. Many may wonder, *What can some therapist tell me?*
- **Twenty-nine percent don't have enough money or insurance to pay for treatment.**
  This is a very real problem. Treatment for depression can be expensive, and it can seem impossible to find adequate care without insurance. Most people, however, do have access to community mental health centers, training facili-

ties, or teaching hospitals, where good care can be found at a reasonable cost.

- **Seventeen percent would be too afraid to seek help.**

Fear can be paralyzing, but knowledge can break the grip of fear. Most people who are too afraid to seek help do not know what kind of help is available. They may have visions of being locked away in a psychiatric hospital or being drugged, shocked, or operated upon. Thankfully, we have learned a lot about treating mental illnesses in the last few decades, and these kinds of images are now strictly for the movies.

- **Seventeen percent said they don't know enough about available treatments or about depression itself.**

This obstacle to treatment is the easiest to overcome. Arming yourself with knowledge about the causes of and treatments for depression is the best way to overcome fear and ensure that you will get the best care available. Understanding what is happening to you and learning to take an active role in your treatment increases your chances of overcoming depression and learning to manage this often chronic illness.

- **Twelve percent said feelings of hopelessness would keep them from getting help.**

Hopelessness is a pervasive symptom of depression. It can be terribly difficult to convince someone who sees no hope for the future that they can be helped. We cannot stress this enough: The great majority of people suffering from depression *can* be helped. The future does not have to be as painful as the present.

- **Sixty percent believe prayer and faith will successfully treat depression "almost all of the time" or "some of the time."**

Faith and prayer are our strength. They are the foundation of our communities, our families, and our personal well-being. African Americans' legendary faith in a higher power and greater purpose has kept us whole and helped us thrive despite countless assaults on our humanity. It only makes sense that we would turn to God when we are depressed. But depression cannot be cured by faith alone. Strong faith can certainly help the healing process, and it can bring us out of minor cases of the blues. It can give us reason to live (several of the women we interviewed told us that their faith kept them from taking their lives). If you believe in a compassionate God, then you will know that He does not want you to suffer.

Even though depressive episodes usually end on their own in six months or so, without treatment they are likely to recur, and subsequent episodes are likely to be more severe. Without appropriate treatment, clinical depression will continue to insinuate itself into all aspects of your life, straining your relationships, jeopardizing your job, and perhaps ultimately killing you. Treating depression is crucial. It saves families, relationships, jobs, and lives.

Fear of Treatment: The History of Blacks and the Medical Establishment

One reason many of us don't seek treatment for depression (and many other illnesses) is our well-founded distrust of the medical establishment. Though the Tuskeegee Experiment (see the box on page 162) is the best-known example of medical abuse of African Americans, there are many others. In 1952, Dr. Chester M. Southam of the Sloan-Kettering Institute injected nearly 400 inmates—almost half of them Black—at the Ohio State Prison with live cancer cells as part of an experiment. (Southam almost lost his license for doing the same thing to private patients years later; he was not censured for injecting the prisoners, however). Experiments at the Medical College of Virginia subjected some Black and white patients (including sixty-six children) to radiation burns and injected others with radioactive material to see if Blacks and whites responded differently. In the 1960s and '70s, many Black women who gave birth in some Southern hospitals were sterilized against their will. Often, white physicians have perpetuated derogatory myths about Blacks' alleged stamina and remarkable healing powers. Consequently, we have not received compassionate care. Clearly, we have good reason to be suspicious of doctors and researchers.

Fortunately, as these abuses were exposed, the public put pressure on universities and government research institutes to stop this kind of immoral experimentation. New procedures were put in place to prevent this type of abuse from happening again. Today, medical research cannot be carried out without the informed written consent of the participant. In other words, researchers must explain the purposes and procedures of all studies to participants, who may then opt out of the study at any time with no penalty.

Even so, Blacks still report that medical providers often treat them differently than whites. Some young Black women, for example, have complained that nurses at some family-planning clinics coerce them into getting the controversial contraceptive injection Depo-Provera, but do not offer it to young white women nearly as often. Recent studies have found that Blacks are less likely than whites to receive the most aggressive treatment after a heart attack. For these (good) reasons, some of us will never trust anyone in a lab coat.

Our history is real and cannot be forgotten. We have been hurt. But we cannot allow this history of medical abuse to keep us from getting treatment we need today. There are caring health-care professionals of all ethnicities who can help. Instead, we must become informed health-care consumers. We must go into the doctor's office with our eyes open, well-informed, prepared to ask questions, and confident that we deserve and will demand the best treatment available.

> ## THE TUSKEEGEE SYPHILIS EXPERIMENT
>
> The most infamous case of medical abuse in U.S. history ended less than twenty-five years ago, when journalists exposed the Tuskeegee Syphilis Experiment. The Macon County, Georgia, public health department studied 400 Black men, all infected with syphilis, over a period of forty years. The men were never told that they had syphilis, a sexually transmitted disease that can cause nerve degeneration, blindness, insanity, and, eventually, death. The men were lured into the study with promises of free medical care, though the "care" they received was highly suspect. Researchers drew blood and monitored the effects of the disease, but they never treated the men, even after penicillin, which cures syphilis, was discovered. Many of the men died as a result of the disease; those who survived were permanently disabled. To this day, researchers have not made reparations to the families of those men whose lives were sacrificed in the name of science, though in 1997 President Bill Clinton did finally apologize for the role the U.S. government played in the experiment.

Treating Depression: What Is Appropriate?

Perhaps you are convinced that you need treatment for your depression. Who do you turn to for help? What kind of treatments are available? What works?

These are very important questions. The only thing worse than untreated depression is depression that is treated inappropriately. Unfortunately, confusion and misinformation about treatment abound. The good news is that there are proven treatments for depression, and finding qualified professionals who can provide those treatments may not be as difficult as you might think. We have outlined four important steps that will help you find the most appropriate and effective treatment possible, and get the most out of that treatment:

> **Step 1:** Get a complete physical examination.
> **Step 2:** Know your treatment options.
> **Step 3:** Find a qualified mental health professional to work with.
> **Step 4:** Learn to be an active partner in your own healing.

There are several approaches to treating depression, and many types of professionals are qualified to provide those treatments. Following these steps will increase your chances of finding treatment that works for you.

While we believe that this kind of step-by-step approach to finding treatment is best, we also recognize that it requires an amount of energy and initiative some depressed people just don't have. If you are (or someone you care about is) so severely depressed that following these steps proves too difficult (for example, you can't get out of bed all day or you can't concentrate on anything for more than a few minutes), see your primary care doctor or a psychiatrist (call a local teaching hospital—one affiliated with a university—or outpatient psychiatric clinic to find a psychiatrist). **If you are feeling suicidal, call 911 and go to the nearest hospital emergency room. Suicidal feelings are a medical emergency. Do not wait for suicidal feelings to go away.**

Step One: Get a Complete Physical Examination.
Why is a physical exam important if depression is a mental illness? First, as mentioned in chapter 7, there are many medical illnesses that look like depression—that is, they cause de-

pressive symptoms. For example, hypothyroidism, caused by an underactive thyroid gland, is a widespread ailment among Black women, and it is one of the most common causes of depressive symptoms. Symptoms of hypothyroidism include loss of appetite and energy, insomnia, and sad or depressed mood—the same as clinical depression. Hypothyroidism can be easily treated with medication, and once the condition is corrected, the depressive symptoms disappear.

Also, prescription and over-the-counter medications may be to blame for your depressive symptoms. Medication for high blood pressure and heart disease—conditions that affect a great number of Black women—commonly cause depressive symptoms. Even some often-used painkillers can cause depressive symptoms.

A complete physical exam will help determine whether any medical illnesses or drug reactions are at the root of your depression. If a physical illness or drug reaction is to blame for your symptoms, treating the illness or changing or stopping the medication should relieve them. Furthermore, if your depressive symptoms do have a physical cause, it can be very important to treat the physical illness as soon as possible. Depression is frequently the first symptom of a serious medical condition like cancer or heart disease. If your depressive symptoms are caused by such an illness, treating the depression with antidepressant drugs or therapy is not likely to work, and it will allow the underlying illness to worsen.

Step Two: Know Your Treatment Options
There are two main forms of treatment for depression: psychotherapy (also known as talk therapy) and drug treatment (pharmacotherapy). As with the causes of depression, disagreements over which form of treatment is best are common. Biopsychiatrists and other medical doctors insist that medication is all that is needed to treat depression, from the mildest case to

MEDICAL CONDITIONS AND MEDICATIONS
THAT CAN CAUSE DEPRESSIVE SYMPTOMS

Medical Conditions

Before your doctor confirms a diagnosis of major depression, dysthymia, or any other depressive illness, he or she will want to rule out the possibility that any of the following conditions are causing your depressive symptoms.

- Stroke
- Dementia (including Alzheimer's disease)
- Infections
- HIV
- Syphilis
- Mononucleosis
- Pneumonia
- Tuberculosis
- Chronic fatigue syndrome
- Infectious hepatitis
- Autoimmune disorders such as rheumatoid arthritis, lupus, and multiple sclerosis
- Narcolepsy
- Epilepsy
- Parkinson's disease
- Huntington's disease
- Cancer
- Heart disease
- Thyroid, parathyroid, and adrenal gland disorders

Black women are at greater risk for developing many of these conditions, especially stroke, heart disease, lupus, and certain cancers. It is particularly important that your doctor rule out any illnesses or conditions that disproportionately affect Black women or that run in your family.

We are also at greater risk for HIV infection and other

sexually transmitted diseases. Make sure you are tested for STDs and HIV if you are at risk (for instance, if you have more than one sex partner, if your partner has multiple partners, or if you use IV drugs).

Medications

All medications have unwanted side effects, and depression is a common side effect of many prescription and over-the-counter drugs. Some of the most commonly used ones are:

- Ibuprofen (Advil, Nuprin, and Motrin)
- Antibiotics (including ampicillin, streptomycin, and tetracycline)
- Antihypertensive (high blood pressure) drugs and drugs for heart disease (like the beta-blockers Inderal and Lopressor; alpha-metyldopa, clonidine, digitalis, lidocaine, reserpine, and diuretics or water pills)
- Sedatives and hypnotics (including barbiturates like Valium and benzodiazepines)
- Gastrointestinal medication (Tagamet)
- Amphetamines
- Diet pills
- Oral contraceptives (the Pill)
- Illicit drugs (including marijuana, cocaine, heroin, and PCP)

Be sure to tell your doctor if you take any of the above drugs. If you take a number of medications, making a list of all the drugs you take might be helpful for both you and your doctor. If that seems too complicated, just gather up your medications and take them to the doctor with you.

the most severe. Some psychologists and other psychotherapists argue that drugs are the easy way out, that they are simply a crutch for people who don't want to face their problems head-on.

Most clinicians who treat depression fall between these two extremes. They recognize that antidepressant drugs are often necessary to relieve the symptoms of depression, and therapy is necessary to get at the psychological issues that contribute to depression and to help the depressed person regain self-esteem and repair damaged relationships. We discuss psychotherapy, drug therapy, and other treatments for depression in detail in chapters 8 and 9.

Step Three: Find a Qualified
Mental Health Professional

Even when we do decide to seek treatment for depression, we are often confused as to who can really help us. Few African Americans actually see professionals who are truly qualified to treat the illness. According to the National Mental Health Association survey:

- Twenty-seven percent of African-American respondents said they would seek treatment from their family doctor if they suffered from depression.
- Twenty-seven percent would handle it by themselves.
- Nineteen percent would consult family or friends.
- Fourteen percent would go to a psychiatrist or counselor.
- Twelve percent would go to a minister or priest.
- Three percent wouldn't know what to do.

Although some family doctors are well-versed in treating depression, the majority are not. In fact, as mentioned earlier, family practitioners fail to diagnose depression in half of their patients who have it. Nor is everyone who calls himself or herself a therapist really qualified to treat depression. Although ministers, priests, family, and friends are wonderful and necessary support for the depressed person, they cannot treat the illness. (Some ministers or priests who have special training as pastoral counselors might be qualified to treat depression, however; see below). Self-help techniques are empowering and extremely helpful for many depressed people, but self-help is not the same as treatment.

So who can treat depression? How do you find a mental health professional who is qualified? Getting the best treatment may require a little detective work. You will also need to decide what approach to treatment seems best for you. Do you want to see someone who can prescribe medication if you need it? Do you think psychotherapy is the best place to start? You should consider how race and gender may affect your treatment, as well. Is seeing a Black woman important to you, or are you equally comfortable with seeing a man or a woman, a Black therapist or a white one? These are all important things to think about.

You should also know your doctor's or therapist's educational background. Not all mental health professionals have the same training or the same theoretical view of depression. As a result, different professionals approach treatment in very different ways. It is up to you to decide what approach feels most comfortable. You can make a more informed decision as to what type of mental health professional to see if you know the differences between them.

Types of Mental Health Professionals.
Psychiatrists are medical doctors (M.D.'s) who specialize in treating mental illness. Their education includes four years of medical school plus at least three years of residency training in psychiatry. Since they are mental health specialists, psychiatrists are more likely to keep on top of the latest advances in treating

depression than the average family doctor. Some psychiatrists use psychotherapy as their primary (or only) approach to depression; others, such as biopsychiatrists, treat the illness with medication alone (though they will usually work with a psychotherapist if therapy is needed). Some routinely use both approaches. Psychiatrists are the only mental health professionals who can prescribe medication for depression.

Psychologists are mental health professionals who treat mental and emotional disorders with verbal psychotherapy. Doctoral-level psychologists have either Ph.D. or Psy.D. degrees; both complete four years of course work in clinical psychology, several years of practicum training in psychotherapy, and a one-year therapy internship. (The main difference between the two is that Ph.D.'s have more training in research and a Psy.D.'s training is primarily clinical).

Masters-level psychologists (M.A.'s or M.S.'s) complete two years of graduate school in psychology. Master's-level psychologists who provide psychotherapy are usually supervised by Ph.D's or Psy.D.'s. Doctoral-level psychologists can become licensed (or registered) clinical psychologists. Licensed clinical psychologists complete a certain number of hours of supervised clinical experience after completing their degree and before taking a licensing exam. In most states, only doctoral-level psychologists can sit for the licensing exam or go into private practice.

Clinical social workers are mental health professionals who have completed a graduate program in social work. This training includes course work in social welfare issues, human development, psychology, and psychotherapy with two years of field work, which includes psychotherapy training. At the end of their training, they earn a masters of social work (M.S.W.) degree. Licensed clinical social workers (LCSWs or LICSWs) have at least two years of experience beyond the degree and have passed a licensing examination. Many of the therapists in managed-care organizations like HMOs are licensed clinical social workers. LCSWs and LICSWs can legally provide private practice psychotherapy.

Psychiatric nurses can also provide psychotherapy. Psychiatric nurses have either master's degrees or Ph.D.'s in nursing, plus experience in psychotherapy (often in hospital settings).

Pastoral counselors are ministers or priests who have special training in counseling or psychotherapy. Some have dual M.Div. (master's of divinity) and M.S.W. degrees; some have counseling degrees; and others have simply attended a training program in pastoral counseling. Though they may be wonderful counselors, not all ministers or priests are qualified to treat depression; in fact, relatively few are. If you would be most comfortable seeing a religious person for treatment, ask your minister or priest if he or she can recommend a clergy member who has training and experience in treating depression. There are also many psychiatrists, psychologists, and clinical social workers for whom faith and religion are a big part of their approach to treatment, though they are not ministers or priests. If religion or spirituality is very important to you, you might want to look for a therapist who describes himself or herself as a Christian therapist (depending on where you live, you may also be able to find therapists of other faiths who use their religion in their work).

Psychotherapists/counselors: People who simply call themselves psychotherapists or counselors may be trained as psychologists, social workers, or counselors, or they may have no training at all. If you are considering seeing someone who describes himself or herself as a psychotherapist or counselor, check carefully and determine what kind of education and training he or she has. Unfortunately, there are many unqualified people who call themselves therapists. Spending your time and money on someone who is not qualified to help you means living with depression longer than you have to.

FINDING A QUALIFIED MENTAL HEALTH PROFESSIONAL

Finding someone qualified to treat depression can be daunting, but don't give up hope. Here are some suggestions for locating professionals with experience in treating depression.

- Ask your primary-care doctor for a referral (you will have to do this if you are a member of an HMO). If you are not in an HMO, your internist or family practitioner is a good place to start.
- Ask a friend or family member if she knows of any good therapists or psychiatrists. Maybe you think no one you know would ever see a mental health professional, but you never know. Of course, if you don't feel comfortable asking someone you know, don't do it. There are many other ways to find help.
- If your job has an employee assistance program (EAP), ask for a confidential evaluation with an EAP counselor. The counselor can then make a referral to a qualified mental health provider.
- Ask your priest or minister. Many churches have health ministries.
- Call or write a professional organization. The organizations listed in chapter 13 can give you the names of several professionals in your area.
- Call a teaching hospital (one associated with a university) and ask if they have a depressive disorders clinic. Many universities have low-cost clinics staffed by graduate students who are supervised by experienced psychiatrists or psychologists. Some universities can also refer you to private practitioners who graduated from their program.
- Call a local women's health center. Most can refer you to therapists in your area; some have therapists on staff.
- Call a local community mental health center.

Step Four: Learn to Be an Active Partner
in Your Own Healing

When you are depressed, you may not have the energy to do much more than pick up the telephone and make an appointment with a doctor or therapist. That's OK. Just making an appointment is the first step in taking responsibility for your health.

Once you have made the appointment, it is up to you to get the most you can out of your treatment. It may take a while for you to feel as if you have any control over what is happening to you, but try to keep in mind that you do. Eventually, you will come out of your depression. In the meantime, try to be an active partner in your healing. Being an active partner means:

- Going to your doctor's and therapy appointments on time, even when you don't feel like it.
- Being totally honest with your doctor or therapist. Don't hold back anything—*nothing*.
- Learning as much as you can about depression; read books, check out videos from the local health library.
- Becoming an expert about any medication prescribed for your depression.
- Taking your medication as prescribed.
- Making time for yourself and doing good things for yourself.
- Telling people in your life that you need time for yourself.
- Taking care of other aspects of your health (eating right, exercising, getting treatment for any other health problems you have).
- Not doing anything that makes you feel uncomfortable.
- Clearing your life of toxic people, situations, and places. This may be easier said than done. If you can't, for instance, get away from family members that put too many

demands on you, make a plan to manage their demands. Work on it with your therapist or with an understanding friend. If your job is too stressful, think about ways you could make it less stressful, or try to come up with other things you'd like to do. You have more control over your life than you might think.

- Surrounding yourself with people who love and respect you.
- Learning how to say no.
- Believing that you are worth taking care of.

9

· · · · · · ·

The Talking Cure:
Psychotherapy for Depression

For many of us, the idea of psychotherapy is pretty foreign. Most Black people are not accustomed to using mental health services. Consequently, we may not think about using a psychotherapist when we are having difficulties in our lives. In fact, when someone suggests that we consult a psychotherapist to help us with some problem we are having, our typical response is something like, "I don't want anyone getting into my head," or "What is he or she going to tell me that I don't already know?" Often, we are put off by the idea of telling our business to someone, and we really dislike the idea of *paying* to talk to someone. If you press the issue, people are quick to tell you that they have plenty of people they can talk to—girl-friends, relatives, parents, beauticians, coworkers, a host of people.

Clearly, there are many people to whom we can turn when we have problems, but in reality, none of our social relationships offers the unique qualities that a relationship with a psychotherapist offers—and it is these qualities that are curative.

The relationship with a psychotherapist is a private, confidential relationship in which the sole purpose is the well-being of the client or patient. In important respects, it is a skewed, one-sided relationship, and the most important person in the relationship is the client. So, if the therapist is having a bad hair day, financial woes, a headache, or boyfriend blues, the client is not burdened with any of this. In many ways, the therapist's feelings don't matter one bit. The therapist is available for the client to assist her in resolving the difficulties that brought her into therapy.

Of course, social relationships are not constructed this way. Social relationships necessarily involve a high degree of mutuality and reciprocity, and they exist for the well-being of both parties. If you are in need of comfort in a social relationship, you are expected to make that need known and the other person in the relationship is expected (appropriately) to consider your needs.

The chief advantage of the one-sided psychotherapy relationship is that for a change, you have the opportunity to talk about your concerns with impunity. Additionally, since the therapist is not familiar with anything about you except what you are capable of sharing with him or her at the moment, it is an objective view of you in a relationship centered around your psychological reality. Now, what is this *psychological reality*? It is the world according to you; it is life viewed through your lenses; life as experienced and defined by you. This is a crucial point for ultimately, your perceptions—your psychological reality—contribute to both your pain and your improvement.

For example, we all know of instances where people insist that things are proceeding far more terribly than objective reality suggests. They experience seemingly minor inconveniences as insurmountable obstacles; a setback is a death sentence and a bad stint is synonymous with chronic misery. From the outside (objective reality view), the person is having a bad spell. From the person's psychological reality, life is an unbearable necessity that the person feels ill equipped to manage. It is this reality that is the central focus of psychotherapy.

To be sure, depending on the therapist's perspective, this reality will be responded to in different ways. But this reality is the key factor in helping the patient or client in psychotherapy, and all efforts are made to help her work with her idiosyncratic reality.

Though antidepressants are the first-line treatment for severe depressions (especially if you have a lot of physical symptoms or if you are suicidal), treating mild cases of depression with drugs is generally not necessary. Even more severe cases can respond to therapy, especially when combined with antidepressant medication. In recent years, psychiatry has relied heavily on the use of antidepressant medications to treat depression. There seem to be several reasons for this. The development of drugs like Prozac has brought enormous relief, and these drugs have posed few risks for users. Also, changes in the health care system have endorsed any treatment that is safe, efficacious, and quick. Pills work faster than words, and depressive symptoms abate quickly in some cases. However, despite the enthusiastic use of medications, outpatient office psychotherapy is still an optimal choice for the treatment of most depressions. Therapy can help resolve issues that are related to the cause of the depression, and those that arise as a result of the depression, such as problems in relationships, at work, or with self-concept and self-esteem. Therapy is essential in helping people develop better coping and stress management strategies. Therapy is the obvious treatment of choice for people who are unable to take antidepressant medications for health reasons or because they are strongly opposed to taking medications.

Celeste is one of many depressed Black women who has been helped by psychotherapy:

> *Just talking to my therapist helps me, because I can talk about how I'm feeling without it being overwhelming, like it*

*is with my mother or somebody close to me. I think it is good
to have somebody who doesn't have the emotional attachment
to you that family and friends do, and so doesn't feel guilty
about me feeling so bad. I can just talk. And as I talk, I've
had a lot of lightbulbs go off and a lot of awareness of why
things happen a certain way. Things about myself . . . why
I made the choices I made. That helps me.*

Types of Psychotherapy

Various types of therapy are used in the treatment of depression. The three most commonly used are psychodynamic therapy, cognitive therapy, and interpersonal therapy. Each form of therapy was developed from the corresponding theory of psychological well-being and illness. Accordingly, cognitive therapy works to help the depressed woman change maladaptive, self-defeating thoughts. Psychodynamic therapy works to help the depressed woman gain insight into the underlying reasons that impede her functioning. Interpersonal therapy draws on these as well as other approaches. Let's look more closely at how depression is addressed from each perspective.

Psychodynamic Psychotherapy

Psychodynamic psychotherapy is the offspring of psychoanalysis. Psychoanalysis is an intensive form of outpatient psychotherapy that helps the patient look very closely at the realtionship betweeen the events that transpired in her early life and current problems. The patient sees the analyst (a psychotherapist who is trained in the techniques and theory of psychoanalysis) four to five times per week, for forty-five or fifty minutes each visit, for anywhere from four to six years. The time spent with the analyst is unstructured and the patient discusses whatever she wants. The analyst makes interpretations that help the patient connect the things she is talking about with her current problems.

How it works. Psychodynamic psychotherapy is, in most opinions, considerably more practical than psychoanalysis. The patient is seen by a psychotherapist who is trained in the principles of psychodynamic theory and who has developed some expertise in psychodynamic psychotherapy. The patient is often seen one or two times a week. She sits and faces the therapist. Much like psychoanalysis, the emphasis is on understanding the relationship between events that occurred early in life and current problems. Like psychoanalysis, an assumption of psychodynamic therapy is that we have ready access to some thoughts (conscious material) and remote access to other thoughts (unconscious material) that may profoundly affect our functioning. The unconscious material has an important impact on our actions, and deciphering and understanding unconscious feelings is an important part of the healing process. The second assumption is that problematic patterns tend to repeat over time. Therefore, if the therapist closely observes the interactions between herself and the client, she can gather data about the kinds of difficulties likely to emerge in the patient's life. Such material is interpreted back to the patient. The insight gathered from this interpretation/ explanation and the subtle but significant perceptual shifts that accompany these insights promote growth.

What to expect. During the initial visit with the psychodynamic psychotherpist, be prepared to talk at length about yourself. The therapist will make an effort to establish some initial rapport and will ask you to discuss your symptoms, their intensity and duration, and the ways they impact your life. She will want to know about other aspects of your current life: your work, family life, friendships, and intimate relationships. As you can imagine, this is a lot of information, and the forty-five or fifty minutes pass very quickly. Often, the time will end before anything definitive can be said about the depression.

(Obviously, if you are so incapacitated that you are unable to speak and someone else has accompanied you to the session, you will be referred to a psychiatrist or other medical doctor for a medication assessment). If you are able to come in without assistance and talk about your concerns, the therapist will probably invite you back in the next two or three days to complete the diagnostic assessment.

The second and third visit will be spent looking more closely at your symptoms, your current life, and the feelings you have about the events transpiring in your life. You will also look at your feelings about and reactions to the way things are going in therapy. While some or none of this might seem directly related to the reasons you consulted the therapist, she is trying to determine whether there are correlations between the current depression and long-standing issues related to your early life. She may even ask you about dreams, nightmares, recurring fantasies, etc.

Usually around the fourth visit, the psychodynamic psychotherapist feels she is in a position to offer an initial formulation or impression about how she understands your depression. She proposes a treatment plan outline, though she cautions that much of what happens in psychodynamic psychotherapy is unpredictable and dependent on what emerges over the course of treatment.

The therapist will urge you to speak freely and not to censor anything you think and want to say. She will stress that the tools for treatment are your words, for your words provide her with access to your feelings, which are the key to resolving the issues that contribute to the depression. She will caution that you might discover things that you had not anticipated and that you might actually feel worse prior to feeling better. She will reassure you that psychodynamic psychotherapy is a process and that things may seem vague and unsettling long before they seem clear and helpful.

Pros and cons. Some people consider the unstructured, open-ended format of psychodynamic psychotherapy a disadvantage. They feel the patient is allowed to wander all over the place with no sense of direction. Some people argue that the process is long, and that more efficient forms of treatment exist. Still others feel that Black people think too concretely to participate in such a highly abstract form of treatment.

While psychodynamic psychotherapy is unstructured, meaning the therapist does not decide what is going to be discussed, the work typically organizes itself around one or two salient themes that develop from the patient's discussions. It is worth noting that unstructured does not mean chaotic or disorganized. An assumption of psychodynamic psychotherapy is that people discuss what they need to discuss or are psychologically able to discuss at any given time. Therefore, everything is considered important and it is the job of the therapist to understand how these things contribute to the illness.

Until fairly recently, the conventional wisdom was that African Americans were not suitable candidates for psychodynamic psychotherapy. Psychodynamic therapy requires a high level of tolerance for frustration and delayed gratification, as well as a capacity for abstract reasoning and self-reflection. Many made the racist assumption that Blacks were simply not sophisticated enough to benefit from this type of therapy. They wrongly believed that we were simple, concrete-thinking folks who needed a more directive, problem-solving approach. Although it is true that psychodynamic therapy does not work for everyone (for example, it is most effective with people who are very verbal, who are comfortable opening up about very personal issues, and who value insight and introspection), these differences have to do with personality and communication styles, not with race.

Though therapy is ultimately a healing process, it can be difficult. Some women face down devastating memories of abuse or loss in therapy. Others find that they must let go of long-held views of significant others—or themselves—that just don't ring true. Psychodynamic therapy can really shake your foundations. For this reason, some people believe this type of therapy is most useful when you have started to come out of a depression, not when you are in the thick of it. But a skilled therapist will be able to work with you at any stage of your depression, provided you are able to talk about your feelings and experiences. (Antidepressant medication is usually recommended for people who are severely depressed—those with marked physical symptoms and who are unable to talk about their feelings. Once the severe symptoms have lifted somewhat, therapy is usually very helpful.)

The length of time of treatment with psychodynamic therapy varies. Because depression affects so many aspects of your life, the therapy is directed not only at alleviating the symptoms of the depression but at discussing other problems that have developed as a result of it (such as professional, interpersonal, financial, and social problems). So, while it may be possible to get symptom relief in six weeks of therapy, there are often many other matters that need to be discussed before you feel that life is back to normal. Ideally, a depressed woman might see a psychodynamic therapist twice a week for the first six weeks, once a week for about twenty weeks, and once every two weeks for another twenty to twenty-six weeks. Such a course of treatment would take about a year. With managed care, however, there are fewer options for long-term treatment. Some companies only allow six to eight sessions; most will pay for about twenty. As a result, short-term (six to twelve weeks) psychodynamic therapies are becoming more popular.

Contrary to what you may have heard, psychodynamic therapy is not about blaming Mama. Healing occurs through acknowledging past experiences that may have been hurtful or damaging, understanding how those experiences play themselves out in your life now, assimilating that knowledge, and using it to improve self-esteem and current relationships. Good therapists do not encourage their clients to blame others for their problems; instead, they help clients take responsibility for their own well-being.

Cognitive Therapy

Cognitive theory holds that depression is the result of negative, distorted thinking patterns, so the goal of cognitive therapy is to correct those thinking patterns. Depressed women often struggle with thoughts like, *I can't do anything right,* or *All my decisions are bad,* or *Everything that goes wrong in my life (and my children's, partners', or friends' lives) is my fault.* (Think back to Celeste's and Elaine's belief that they always made bad choices.) The aim of cognitive therapy is to help you see the errors in this way of thinking and find more constructive, positive ways of looking at your world.

How it works. Cognitive therapy is time-limited, usually lasting ten to twenty sessions. Sessions run about fifteen to twenty minutes each. During the sessions, the therapist helps you recognize your negative thinking patterns and figure out whether what you are thinking is really true. She does this by using exploratory questioning techniques. For example, you may think, *I am not worthy of unconditional love. If I do not sacrifice myself for others, no one will love me.* This thought reflects your low self-esteem and may foster self-defeating behavior like ignoring your own needs, leading to frustration and anger and fueling your depression. The cognitive therapist would help you decide whether this thought is valid— whether being loved is actually dependent on how much you sacrifice for others in your life. You would come to see that this is a distorted thought that is causing you to behave in a self-defeating way, and that this is contributing to your depression. You would learn how to recognize such erroneous cognitions and change them before they set off a chain of negative thoughts and behavior.

The cognitive therapist works with you to set goals for the therapy. The two of you decide what types of homework assignments and exercises will help you recognize and challenge your distorted negative beliefs. For example, you might keep a journal or thought log of negative thoughts and the situations that provoked them. You would learn how to recognize and restructure these faulty thoughts and assumptions so you could cope better in the future. You might also do role-plays during the therapy sessions, and you might be taught certain assertiveness, problem-solving, or relaxation skills.

Pros and cons. Many studies have found cognitive therapy to be effective in treating depression, and it is often recommended by primary care doctors and psychiatrists as an adjunct to antidepressant medication or for people who refuse to take medication. Cognitive therapy is very focused on the here and now. It does not probe your early life experiences or delve into your unconscious drives and desires. For these reasons, it may be more effective than psychodynamic therapies for those who are more severely depressed, who are uncomfortable with the idea of psychodynamic therapy, or who cannot afford (or whose insurance will not cover) longer-term therapies. However, while this focus on current symptoms and thought patterns can help alleviate depressive symptoms, it cannot get at deeper psychological issues that may contribute to depression. Cognitive therapy is not useful in helping you work on those problems your depression may have caused, either. For some women, cognitive therapy might be useful while in the throes of depression, but more psychodynamically oriented therapy might be necessary once the depressive episode has passed.

Interpersonal Psychotherapy

Interpersonal therapy, or IPT, is not a new form of psychotherapy. Rather, it is a way of applying some of the principles of both psychodynamic and cognitive therapies that has been show to work very well in treating depression. Like cognitive therapy, interpersonal therapy stresses the present. IPT focuses on your social network and current relationships—your interactions with family, friends, coworkers, and community. But like psychodynamic therapy, IPT does look at past experiences to explain current feelings and behavior. The interpersonal approach assumes two things: first, that problems in current relationships are probably rooted in early dysfunctional relationships; and that problems in your current relationships contribute to your depressive symptoms.

How it works. Treatment with IPT usually lasts twelve to sixteen weeks. In once-weekly sessions, you work on changing the behaviors that lead to problems in your relationships (such as guilt and lack of assertiveness). In the first two sessions, the therapist will ask you about your symptoms and about the circumstances related to the onset of the depression. She will try to determine what interpersonal issues seem to be related to the depression. If you are severely depressed and incapacitated, she may recommend a medical consultation for possible medication. The therapist will also begin to think about a therapeutic strategy (what issues should be addressed in future sessions, what skills you may need to work on, etc.). During the middle phase of treatment, the therapist will encourage you to explore these issues and the feelings they engender. You may look at how you communicate with others in your life and work on improving communication skills. Some cognitive techniques may be used to help you overcome negative thought patterns that hamper your relationships, but the focus is always on your interactions with others in your life. The therapist may also use role playing or may contract with you to perform certain tasks. She may also provide you with educational materials and information that will help you better understand your depression.

IPT has been found to alleviate the symptoms of depression quickly. Some women find that treatment with IPT is useful when they are in the acute stages of depression, while psychodynamic therapy helps them deal with issues of abuse and loss once the depression lifts.

What Makes a Good Therapist?

There is no one thing that makes one therapist better than another. Each therapist has his or her own style, so you may have to shop around to find one with whom you feel comfortable. Once you have gotten a few referrals (see chapter 13), call several therapists and ask them the questions listed below. Most therapists will schedule an interview appointment with you, as well. This appointment is a no-commitment opportunity to see if you and the therapist feel as if you can work together. Therapy is a partnership; your comfort level with your therapist is very important. If a therapist makes you feel uneasy or if you do not like his or her style, you will not get as much out of the therapy as you could otherwise.

Questions to Ask

- What is your educational background?
- How long have you been practicing?
- How do you treat depression?
- How do you feel about medication for depression?
- Do you work with/refer your clients to a psychiatrist for medication if necessary?
- What are your fees? Do you have a sliding scale for people who can't pay your full fee?
- What is your cancellation policy?
- Are you familiar with/comfortable with working with African-American clients?

If you are not happy with the answers you get to any of these questions, call the next person on your list. If you feel as if you are interrogating the people you call, don't. Shopping around for a therapist is normal and expected. It is very important that you and the therapist are a good fit. Don't be intimidated.

Race, Gender, and Therapy

For some Black women, the race of their therapist is of primary importance. For others, race makes no difference whatsoever. It is up to you to decide whether the race of your therapist matters.

Historically, all psychotherapists were trained using a Western model of psychology that assumed the white, middle-class way of looking at and living in the world was healthy, and anything else was deviant. While most schools that train therapists have by now recognized the racism inherent in this way of thinking, not all therapists have changed the way they view Black clients. Some still believe our cultural differences are somehow wrong and in need of correction. Some are heavily influenced by stereotypes of African Americans and have trouble seeing Black clients as individuals. Others simply don't have experience in working with Black clients, and may not understand the complex ways in which prejudice and racism color our world.

At the same time, not all Black therapists are comfortable working with all Black clients. We have our prejudices against each other, too. Some Black therapists make judgments about their Black clients because of differences in class background. Others may have skin-color issues that could come into play with Black clients. Good therapists are aware of these feelings when they come up in therapy, and they know how to work them through. However, if such issues arise and make you uncomfortable, be sure to tell your therapist. If they can't be resolved, you may need to find someone else.

You should not feel as if you *should* see a Black therapist if that is not important to you. There is nothing wrong with seeing a therapist of another race. But you should be certain that whomever you choose has experience working with Black clients, and that you feel as if you can open up to him or her without being misunderstood or judged because of your race.

Celeste has been seeing a white male psychologist and is fairly happy with that relationship. She was referred to him through the employee assistance program at her job.

> *Sometimes it's hard to judge therapy and therapists because there is no magic cure. It's not like when you break a leg and then they fix it; they can't measure things that way. I don't have an expectation of a miraculous cure. I know that this is a process and it will take time to heal, to do a lot of things that I've been through.*
>
> *I feel comfortable with my therapist. I feel I can be honest and talk about things. I think I would have preferred a Black female. But he's nearby and when I first started going to him, I thought, "I'm going to switch. I'm just doing this temporarily." But I guess I feel comfortable enough that I didn't. I feel like I have made some progress. I feel like I have a lot more insight into things.*
>
> *I think he understands [racial differences] on some level or I wouldn't be sitting there talking to him. With any white person, you wonder how much they really understand what a Black person is going through. But we talk about some of those things.*
>
> *I'm satisfied with that therapeutic relationship because I'm getting something out of it for myself. Most of the work, I feel, gets done outside the therapy, you know. A lot of my aha's and my thoughts go off when I'm not sitting in there.*

For Maya, her therapist's race was not as important as her understanding of sexuality issues.

> *I've been off and on in therapy from the time I was in high school. I had hooked up with a nonprofit organization that helped high school kids. I had this Black woman therapist—I specifically requested a woman therapist because I didn't think a man would understand what I was saying about some of the stuff that was going on in my relationships with the female members of my family. I had this young Black woman who could handle everything but the fact that I was lesbian. And on a regular basis, she tried messing with my head about that. She would say things like, "How do you know that you are a lesbian?" Out of the blue—we would be talking about something else and finally I just confronted her and said, "You know, I think what's really going on is that you have a problem with my being a lesbian. I do not have a problem with my being a lesbian. I'm not going to tolerate it anymore." It was the last conversation that we had about lesbianism, so I felt very constricted. Here I am paying a therapist and I can't talk to her about something that is very significant in my life.*
>
> *I didn't know where else to go at that point. The situation got solved for me because she left. Then I got my current therapist, who is a dream walking. She is white. I love her. I have seen her off and on for the last eight or nine years. It's basically a crisis type of therapy. There have been times when I have had these crises and I have come in because I have been experiencing these overwhelming things that have happened. My therapist has been very supportive. She, too, was a bit uncomfortable at first by my lesbianism and we had one conversation in which I basically said, "The last therapist I had, had a real big problem with my being a lesbian. If it is a problem for you, let me know and I'll find*

another therapist." The conversation resolved. Apparently, she took me seriously and she got her own stuff together that maybe she had some prejudices surrounding homosexuality.

Paying for Therapy

Black women often cite cost when listing the reasons why they don't seek psychotherapy. Yes, therapy can be expensive. But how many of us will spend sixty dollars a week at the beauty shop or thirty dollars a week getting our nails done? Sometimes finding the money to pay for therapy is simply a matter of shifting priorities. Your mental health is more important than your hair or your nails. If you can afford to spend a hundred or more dollars a month on personal upkeep, you can afford therapy. If you find a therapist you like but think his or her fees are a little steep, ask about sliding-scale fees. Many private practitioners do not offer a sliding scale, but some do. It can't hurt to ask.

Some of us really don't have the money for therapy, however. If you can't afford weekly therapy sessions with a therapist in private practice, don't give up. Community mental health centers and university-based clinics usually have sliding-scale fees and may charge as little as ten dollars per session.

Your Rights and Responsibilities in Therapy

As we have said, therapy is a healing process. In order to heal, you must feel supported, respected, and listened to in therapy. You should never feel abused, threatened, or coerced. The following is a list of your rights and responsibilities in therapy.

- You have the right to expect complete confidentiality. Your therapist should not discuss your treatment with anyone other than a supervisor (if he or she is in training).

- You have the right to ask the interview questions listed earlier in this chapter, and to expect honest answers.
- You have the right to be an active participant in your treatment. You should be informed of what to expect in treatment before you begin.
- You have the right to refuse to do anything that makes you feel uncomfortable.
- You have the right to stop treatment whenever you want to.
- You should not tolerate feeling mistreated by your therapist. If your therapist often makes you feel put down, defensive, hurt, or mistreated, or if your therapist responds in a way that minimizes your feelings or that feels blameful, get another therapist.
- You have the right to report any inappropriate behavior (including sexual advances) on the part of your therapist to your state licensing board.

How Do You Know
When You're Done with Therapy?

Therapy is a resource to be used whenever and however you need it. It is a process that can be used for crises, or it can be used for sustenance and maintenance. It is often easier to tell when you are done with a crisis-oriented therapy: You're done when the crisis is over. The time-limited or short-term therapies like cognitive and interpersonal therapy have a set number of sessions. The therapist will tell you how many sessions you will have at the outset. If you and the therapist decide that you need more sessions, a limited number will be added.

Being done with more open-ended therapies is highly subjective. Often, the patient and therapist collaborate and conclude that the patient is doing better. They then set a termination date and work toward ending at that time.

Therapy can be a very effective, empowering process. Good

therapy will not only help you out of your depression, it will help you feel more in control of your life. Finding a good therapist and going through the process of healing is one of the best things you can do for yourself.

10

. . . .

Drug Therapies and
Other Treatments for Depression:
The New Frontier?

By some accounts, we have become a Prozac nation, popping the popular antidepressant (as well as many others) as if they were vitamins. But while the rest of America has embraced antidepressants, Black America most decidedly has not. Only 34 percent of African Americans polled in the National Mental Health Association survey said they would take antidepressant medication if their doctor prescribed it.

African Americans have a long, unpleasant history with drugs prescribed for mental illness. Racist assumptions about our intelligence and emotional functioning and a lack of understanding of Black culture have led many clinicians to misdiagnose Blacks who reported symptoms or showed signs of mental illness. For years, most clinicians and researchers assumed that Blacks didn't get depressed—we weren't sophisticated enough. Consequently, we were often diagnosed as psychotic when we were in fact depressed, and we were put on powerful antipsychotic drugs that we did not need. We are suspicious of anyone pushing mind-altering prescriptions our way; we wonder if they are meant to control us and keep us quiet (the fact that research on using drugs to control violence in young Black men has become popular again only strengthens our already healthy suspicion about psychoactive drugs).

Although our reluctance to take antidepressants makes sense, it can mean that we get less than optimal treatment. People with severe depressions may require medication to be able to function at even a minimal level during a depressive episode. Antidepressants can also prevent future episodes or can keep future episodes from becoming severe. Most people, even severely depressed ones, begin to feel much better in a month with medication. The majority of clinicians experienced in treating depression agree that combined treatment with antidepressants and psychotherapy is the most effective approach for moderately to severely depressed patients. If your doctor or therapist has suggested an antidepressant for you, don't dismiss the idea out of hand. Think it over. Medication may be necessary—it may even save your life. But if you decide medication is not for you, remember, no one can force you to take it. You do have the right to refuse.

Antidepressants: An Introduction

Antidepressants have come a long way since they were developed in the 1950s. The first antidepressants, called *MAO inhibitors (monoamine oxidase inhibitors)* were a breakthrough in treating depression, but their numerous side effects—and the fact that patients taking them had to severely restrict their diets to prevent dangerous hypertensive reactions—made them less than ideal. (MAO inhibitors are still used to treat depression in some cases; we will discuss this later in this chapter.) The second generation of antidepressants, the *tricyclics*, had fewer side effects and required no dietary restrictions. Many doctors still use tricyclics as their first line of defense against depression.

The newest class of antidepressant drugs, the *SSRIs (selective serotonin reuptake inhibitors)*—of which Prozac is one—are perhaps the best known and most widely prescribed of the anti-

SYMPTOMS THAT INDICATE MEDICATION MIGHT BE NECESSARY

Not every depressed person needs medication. However, there are certain symptoms that indicate that medication might be necessary. Some of these are:

- Agitation
- Depression that is worse in the morning
- Extreme indecisiveness
- Extreme irritability, angry outbursts, or loss of control
- Hallucinations or delusions
- Inability to get out of bed
- Medication for depression has helped you (or a parent or sibling) before
- Panic attacks (feeling very anxious, fearful, or out of control, and having physical symptoms like heart palpitations, sweating, shortness of breath, chest pains, trembling or shaking, dizziness, and/or nausea)
- Suicidal thoughts

If you have any of these symptoms, you should seriously consider taking medication if your doctor recommends it.

depressants. One reason for their popularity is the fact that they have fewer side effects than tricyclics (especially the potentially dangerous cardiac side effects), though some have raised concerns that they can, in rare cases, cause dramatic (sometimes violent) personality changes. Finally, there are a number of antidepressants that don't belong to any of these classes, and are known as *atypical* antidepressants. These are most often prescribed for patients who do not respond to tricyclics or SSRIs, or who can't tolerate the side effects of those drugs. The wide variety of antidepressants currently available means that if one drug doesn't help you, chances are that another one will.

As discussed in chapter 7, antidepressants work by restoring the balance of certain neurotransmitters, most commonly serotonin, norepinephrine, and dopamine. The various classes of antidepressants do this in different ways. The MAO inhibitors, for example, affect the metabolism of all three of these neurotransmitters, while the SSRIs, as their name implies, act primarily on serotonin. The tricyclics have their greatest effect on norepinephrine, though some also act on serotonin, epinephrine, and dopamine. Some of the atypical antidepressants act primarily on dopamine; others may act on any one or all of these neurotransmitters.

Why is this important? Researchers now believe that a deficiency of one neurotransmitter can cause a different type of depression, or a different symptom profile, than a deficiency of another. They have observed that people who have the classic melancholic symptoms (those who have lost pleasure in all activities, do not feel better when something good happens, have lost a lot of weight, feel extreme guilt, and whose depression is worse in the morning) respond very well to tricyclics but very poorly to MAO inhibitors. Those with atypical depression (who gain weight, sleep a lot, feel that their limbs are heavy or paralyzed, and are extremely sensitive to rejection) tend to respond well to MAO inhibitors. The success of the SSRIs makes researchers think that many people may have serotonin-specific depressions. As a result, by carefully noting your symptoms, your doctor may be better able to prescribe the right medication for you.

Choosing an Antidepressant
Your doctor or psychiatrist should take several factors into account in deciding which antidepressant to prescribe for you:

- **Symptom profile**
- **Safety** (What are the side effects? Do you have any medical conditions that would make one class of antidepressants a bad choice for you? Are there any potential interactions with drugs you take for other medical problems?)
- **Tolerability** (What side effects can you live with? Which would make you stop taking the drug?)
- **Cost** (What can you afford? What will your insurance cover?)

Not all doctors will consider each of these factors when prescribing an antidepressant, however. Some have a favorite drug that they try with all their depressed patients. Many fail to take cost into account. Not all doctors are aware of the fact that a symptom profile can help determine which drugs are most likely to be effective. Primary care doctors (family practitioners, gynecologists, and internists) especially may not be up to date on recent advances in treating depression.

Your insurance coverage may also dictate what drug your doctor will prescribe. If you are covered by an HMO, the plan may not pay for the drug your doctor feels is best for you. HMOs use formularies—lists of drugs that their doctors can prescribe. If a drug isn't on the formulary, your doctor can't prescribe it.

In order to help your doctor choose the best antidepressant for you, you must be completely honest. Tell her all your symptoms, medical conditions, and any drugs you take. Be up front about what side effects you can tolerate: If you don't think you can deal with weight gain or an inhibited sex drive, say so. If the drug your doctor prescribes is too expensive, let her know. It won't do you any good if you can't afford to buy it.

It is also important for you to know as much as possible about the drug (or drugs) you are taking. Make sure you are aware of all the potential side effects of any drug you take. If you experience serious problems, call your doctor immediately.

MEDICATION AND WOMEN IN RECOVERY

"I'm in recovery; the program says I can't take any kinds of drugs, so I can't take antidepressants."

As we know, it is possible be diagnosed with both major depressive disorder and substance abuse or dependence. Depression can coexist with other illnesses. For many of us who are struggling to stay sober and effectively work a program, having a doctor tell us that we need medication to help treat our illness is in direct contradiction to our understanding of what the program teaches. Often, depressed women in recovery anguish at the prospect of putting a drug into their bodies, even if the drug is safe, licit, and sanctioned by the medical community. They fear that they are relying on a pill to cure their problems. We disagree.

Most women who are dependent on alcohol and/or illicit drugs *hate* being drug dependent and have made efforts on their own to kick the habit. The nature of the addiction makes relinquishing the drug a mighty challenge and frequently, in our initial attempts to enter recovery on our own, the drug wins. This can be depressing.

We strongly feel that women diagnosed with major depressive disorder and substance abuse or substance dependence are obvious candidates for antidepressant medications. In order to make an informed recommendation about medications, it is important that your doctor have a clear and complete understanding of your substance usage. She or he must know if you use alcohol or illicit drugs, which drugs, how much you use, and how often you use them. This is one of those times when you have to tell the whole truth and nothing but the truth, because your health—and maybe even your life—depends on it. Consider

> this: Hasin and her colleagues determined that among dually diagnosed patients (those with a diagnosis of major depressive disorder and alcohol dependence), improving the depression *increased* the chances of achieving and sustaining abstinence from alcohol. Treating the depression also reduced the chances of a relapse. These authors concluded, "The status of major depressive disorder appears to have an effect on the course of alcoholism in patients with severe depressive disorders."
>
> If properly prescribed and used, antidepressant medication can be tremendously helpful for depressed, substance-dependent or substance-abusing women.

Antidepressant Classes and Side Effects

All drugs have both good and bad effects, and antidepressants are no different. You and your doctor will have to balance the positive effect of symptom relief with potential side effects in order to find the best antidepressant for you. Knowing what to expect from these medications will help you and your doctor find an antidepressant that will work and one that you will tolerate.

The tricyclic antidepressants. The tricyclics are the largest class of antidepressant medications. While they have a number of side effects, they are less expensive than the newer antidepressants. For this reason, many doctors prefer to start treatment with a tricyclic. They include:

Amitriptyline (Elavil, Endep)
Clomipramine (Anafranil)
Desipramine (Norpramin, Pertofrane)
Doxipine (Adapin, Sinequan)
Imipramine (Tofranil)
Nortriptyline (Aventyl, Pamelor)

Trimipramine (Surmontil)
Protriptyline (Vivactil)

Side effects of amitriptyline, doxipine, imipramine, and trimiprimine:

Frequent side effects:
- Drowsiness
- Dry mouth
- Mild constipation

Occasional side effects:
- Light-headedness
- Dizziness
- Urinary hesitancy
- Severe constipation
- Sweating
- Weight gain of ten pounds
- Increased heart rate (tachycardia)
- Skin rashes
- Blurred vision

Rare Side Effects:
- Memory problems
- Severely blurred vision
- Tremors
- Agitation
- Restlessness or a feeling of needing to be in constant motion

Severe Side Effects:
- Seizures
- Inability to urinate
- Paralysis

- Delirium
- Mania

Side effects of desipramine, nortriptyline, and protriptaline:

Frequent side effects:
- Dry mouth
- Tremors
- Increased heart rate

Occasional side effects:
- Dizziness
- Jitteriness
- Anxiety
- Constipation
- Sweating

Rare side effects:
- Drowsiness
- Skin rashes
- Urinary hesitancy

Severe side effects:
- Seizures
- Memory problems
- Mania

The major drawback to tricyclic antidepressants is they are extremely toxic. Overdosing on tricyclics is extremely dangerous and is often fatal. Some doctors will ask a family member to keep these medications out of the depressed person's reach, and administer them at the appropriate time to prevent suicide attempts.

The selective serotonin reuptake inhibitors (SSRIs). The newest class of antidepressant medications, the SSRIs cause fewer and less frequent side effects than tricyclics. They seem to work as well as the tricyclic drugs, but they are the most expensive of the antidepressants. The drugs that belong to this class are:

>   Fluoxetine (Prozac)
>   Paroxetine (Paxil)
>   Sertraline (Zoloft)

Side effects of fluoxetine:

Frequent side effects:
- Nausea
- Drowsiness
- Anxiety

Occasional side effects:
- Decreased sex drive
- Headaches

Rare side effects:
- Severe weight loss
- Skin rashes
- Gas
- Inability to orgasm
- Weight gain

Severe side effect:
Vomiting

Side effects of paroxitine and sertraline:
These drugs have few side effects. The only notable one is that paroxitine (Paxil) sometimes causes sleepiness.

The MAO Inhibitors. This class of antidepressants has the
most side effects. They can also cause severe adverse reactions
when taken with many over-the-counter drugs. They are useful,
however, for people who do not respond to other antidepressants and for those who have atypical depressions. **MAO
inhibitors should not be given to patients with liver disease,
advanced kidney disease, heart disease, hypertension, asthma,
or chronic bronchitis.** The MAO inhibitors include:

> Isocarboxazid (Marplan)
> Phenelzine (Nardil)
> Tranylcypromine (Parnate)

Side effects:

Frequent side effects:
- Insomnia
- Weight gain
- Postural hypotension
- Decreased sex drive
- Inability to orgasm
- Water retention

Occasional side effects:
- Hypertensive episode (blood pressure rises for a short pe-
  riod of time)
- Daytime drowsiness
- Light-headedness
- Inability to orgasm
- Decreased blood pressure

Rare side effects:
- Sweating

- Dry mouth
- Urinary hesitancy

Severe side effects:
- Fainting
- Liver toxicity
- Hypertensive crisis (a sudden, dramatic, life-threatening rise in blood pressure. Symptoms include a sudden, severe headache, flushing, heart palpitations, eye pain, nausea and vomiting, and sensitivity to light.)
- Cerebrovascular disease or stroke
- Mania

Foods to avoid when taking MAO inhibitors:
- Cheeses with a high or moderate tyramine content, such as boursault, cheddar, Camembert, Gruyere, Stilton, Gouda, and Parmesan (only cottage cheese, ricotta, and cream cheese are known to be truly safe)
- Aged and processed meats (smoked meats, sausages, pickled fish)
- Pickles
- Bean curd (tofu)
- Broad beans (fava beans, broad Italian green beans)
- Asian foods (Chinese, Thai, Japanese, etc.), especially with soy sauce or MSG
- Chocolate and cocoa
- Sour cream
- Yogurt
- Avocado
- Figs, dates, and raisins
- Coffee and other beverages with caffeine
- Beer, wine, and sherry

• Any overprocessed foods, overripe fruits and vegetables, or anything of unknown content (be especially careful in restaurants)

When taking MAO inhibitors, it is best to prepare your own meals, to make sure all produce is fresh, and to cook very simple meals.

Drugs that can cause adverse reactions with MAO inhibitors:
• Amphetamines
• Cocaine and other illegal drugs
• Ritalin
• Novocain
• Many cold medicines and decongestants (those that contain phenylpropanolamine)
• Other antidepressants

Atypical antidepressants. These are mostly newer drugs that don't fall into any of the above categories. They generally cause fewer side effects than tricyclics and MAO inhibitors, and are usually prescribed for patients who do not respond to tricyclics or SSRIs. They include:

Alprazolam (Xanax)
Amoxipine (Asendin)
Bupropion (Wellbutrin)
Maprotiline (Ludiomil)
Nefazodone (Serzone)
Trazodone (Desyrel)
Venlaflaxine (Effexor)

Each of these drugs has a different set of side effects, though most of them produce fewer side effects than the other classes of antidepressant drugs. One exception is Wellbutrin, which causes weight loss in 25 percent of those who take it. There is also a greater risk of seizures with Wellbutrin.

Other Medications for Depression

Even if antidepressants do work for you, you may have a need for other types of drugs for other symptoms associated with your depression. Many depressed people also suffer anxiety or panic attacks, or have trouble sleeping. Antianxiety drugs (also called sedatives or minor tranquilizers) and mood stabilizers are often prescribed to relieve these symptoms. Common antianxiety drugs include:

Ativan (lorazepam)
Centrax (prazepam)
Klonopin (clonazepam)
Librium (chlordiazepoxide)
Serax (oxazepam)
Tranxene (clorazepate)
Valium (diazepam)
Xanax (alprazolam)

The most frequent side effects of these drugs are drowsiness and a general sluggish feeling. Many people worry about becoming dependent on these drugs, but dependence is rare. Buspar (buspirone) does not cause sedation or withdrawal, but does not seem to be as effective as the other antianxiety drugs.

Mood Stabilizers

These drugs are most often used for people who have a history of bipolar disorder (manic-depressive illness), though they also seem to boost the effect of antidepressants. Commonly prescribed mood stabilizers are:

Lithium (lithium carbonate)
Depakene or Depakote (valproic acid)
Klonopin (clonazepam)
Tegretol (carbemazepine)

Lithium is the most commonly prescribed mood stabilizer; the others are generally prescribed only when lithium doesn't work. Lithium can be highly toxic, however, and your blood levels will have to be checked constantly to make sure there isn't too much lithium in your bloodstream.

SELF-HELP FOR COMMON SIDE EFFECTS

The most common antidepressant side effects are constipation, dry mouth, weight gain, and postural hypotension. Here are some suggestions for alleviating some of the discomfort caused by these side effects. If these suggestions do not help, or if the side effects are especially severe, tell your doctor as soon as possible.

Constipation
- Eat more fiber (bran muffins, oat bran cereal, fresh fruits and vegetables, and beans and brown rice are good choices).
- Eat prunes or drink prune juice.
- Drink lots of water.
- Exercise.

Dry Mouth
- Drink lots of water (always have a bottle of water with you wherever you go).
- Suck on sugarless hard candy.
- Ask your doctor or pharmacist to recommend a saliva substitute (these are sprays or drops that moisturize the mouth).

Weight Gain
- Eat a high-fiber, low-fat diet.
- Cut down on your snacking and eat only low-fat snacks like unbuttered, air-popped popcorn, fruits, and vegetables.
- Exercise. Walk for twenty minutes each day; buy an exercise video; ride your bike; join a gym. You don't have to spend money to exercise: Most local park districts offer free exercise classes.

Postural Hypotension
- Don't get up too quickly when you have been sitting.
- Keep your feet elevated when sitting.

Managing Life on Medication

Living with medications is never easy, even when you know they are helping you. At first, you may forget to take your medication, especially if you are on several different ones. You may have to contend with side effects. Others may not understand why you have to take medication at all, and they may even try to make you feel badly about it. It may take several tries before your doctor finds the right medication for you. Also, it may take several weeks before you begin to feel the effects of the medication. Hang in there. Finding the right medication and the right dosage takes time. Don't lose hope just because one drug doesn't work for you.

Keisha, Celeste, and Elaine's experiences with medication are good illustrations of what can happen.

I took Xanax, but I was still having problems. I was still crying every day. I was still losing weight. I would still get panic attacks, but when I got them, I would take the Xanax and that would usually help.

My psychiatrist started switching my medications around. She switched me to Prozac and it didn't work. Then she wanted me to take a psychological test. The results said that I had a thought disorder—that my thoughts were disjointed. Then, she put me on Zoloft and Prolixin, which is an antipsychotic medication (for the thought disorder). Now I am taking Paxil and Prolixin, which seem to be working.

I told my last boyfriend that I was taking medication for depression, and he made me feel like antidepressants were like uppers. He didn't understand what they were. He made me feel like I shouldn't need them. So I probably won't tell the next person I date.

—Keisha

I had been put on a lot of different medications, and nothing worked. I was on Prozac for six months. That didn't do anything. During that six-month period, I was given different things to boost the Prozac; lithium was one them. I was given things to help me sleep because of my insomnia, which was really, really bad. I was falling asleep when I was driving because I was so tired. And nothing really worked, except one antidepressant—trazodone—that was given to me to help me sleep, and it did work. It didn't keep me asleep, but when I woke up, I was able to go back to sleep. My problem was I would wake up at 1:30, 2:00 in the morning, and then I couldn't go to sleep for the rest of the night. With that one, I would still wake up, but I was able to fall asleep again.

—Celeste

I had been taking Wellbutrin, which worked very well. But nobody told me I had to keep taking the medication, so I stopped. I got really depressed again. . . . I had to go back into the hospital. After that, I was put on lithium in addition to the Wellbutrin. I'm also taking medication for my thyroid. [Elaine takes Synthroid for hypothyroidism, as well.] *That combination is working well. I haven't been depressed since I started taking the lithium with the Wellbutrin.*

—*Elaine*

Before you decide your medication isn't working, talk to your doctor. Never stop taking your medication because you feel better, as Elaine did. If your doctor thinks you no longer need medication, he or she will take you off it slowly.

Some depressed people will need to take medication for the rest of their lives. Those who have had recurrent depressions are likely to continue to need medication. Learning that you will need antidepressant drugs for the rest of your life can be traumatic. Talk about your feelings with your doctor, and if you are also in therapy, with your therapist. Don't try to sort out your feelings alone.

Other Treatments for Depression: ECT and Light Therapy

Although antidepressants and other medications work for most depressed people, there are those for whom drugs just don't work. When this happens, many doctors will recommend *electroconvulsive therapy (ECT)*.

ECT was first used to treat depression in the late 1930s. When tricyclic antidepressants were introduced in the 1950s, and lithium in the 1960s, ECT fell out of favor with most psychiatrists. Since that time, ECT has gained a reputation as a barbaric, outdated treatment. Many mental health professionals believe ECT is abusive and should never be used.

However, there are some patients for whom ECT is the therapy of last resort. These patients have been prescribed many types of antidepressants, none of which worked (or worked for only a short time). They may have tried different psychotherapies as well. These are people with severe depressions that nothing else has helped. For them, ECT has some definite advantages. Eighty to 90 percent of those treated with ECT do get better.

While ECT sounds scary, it is a safe and very effective treatment for depression. With ECT, patients are put under general anesthesia and small electrodes are placed on the head. A mild electric current is then run through the electrodes. ECT seems to work by affecting the same neurotransmitters that antidepressants do, but for some reason, it works even when antidepressants don't.

Modern ECT is much safer than it used to be. Side effects of ECT are usually temporary, but they can be significant. They include headaches, memory loss, and confusion. If you have severe depressions and they are not helped by medication, your doctor may recommend ECT. If so, don't dismiss the idea automatically. ECT might be your best hope. The side effects can be troubling, but ECT is only recommended for the most severely depressed patients. For them, some slight amount of memory loss is usually a small price to pay for relief from depression that immobilizes them.

Light therapy is most often recommended for people with seasonal depressions. Patients treated with light therapy (or *phototherapy*) are exposed to full-spectrum light from a special light box for controlled periods of time. This type of therapy does not seem to help other types of depression. This treatment must be administered by a medical doctor in a hospital or office setting. You cannot treat yourself with phototherapy.

When Hospitalization Is Necessary

Severe depressions often require hospitalization, either because the depressed person is a danger to herself (she may attempt suicide) or because her symptoms are so severe that she can no longer take care of herself. Signs that you might need to be hospitalized are:

- You have psychotic symptoms (delusions, hallucinations, paranoia, hearing voices).
- You are making a plan to kill yourself.
- You can't feed, clean, or dress yourself.
- You can't stand being alone.

If your doctor recommends hospitalization, don't fight it. It might save your life. Being in the hospital can be frightening in itself, though. You may find yourself with people who have more severe psychiatric illnesses, and some of their behavior might scare you. The hospital staff may be sensitive and caring, or they may seem cold. While in the hospital, you will likely have to go to therapy groups and participate in other therapeutic activities. Some people get a lot out of these activities, but others find them a waste of time. Nevertheless, if you are in danger of killing yourself, either through suicide or self-neglect, the hospital is the best place for you to be. Celeste found the hospital to be quite unpleasant, but she recognizes that she might not have lived had she not been hospitalized.

> *I didn't look like a typical depressed person, I guess. While I was on the [psychiatric] unit, a lot of people wouldn't shower. I always got up in the morning and showered and put a little makeup on. I tried to participate in the therapy sessions. I had a job. Most of the people were unemployed*

because of the depression. I looked like I was in good shape. People were asking me all the time, "Why are you here?" Staff and other people. They didn't get it. They didn't see. And part of it was me because when I'm at my worst, I look my best, usually, you know. I don't let it show.

I thought the staff was disappointing in a lot of ways. They weren't really helpful. One experience really stood out for me. It was in art therapy. I was doing some artwork for my sons. Because I have two sons, I couldn't just bring back one piece of artwork. I had to have two. I needed about two minutes to finish up and they said that this was the end of the session. So, I figured while everybody was in the supply closet, putting things away, I would just finish up. I was trying to finish up real quick and one of the therapists got really angry at me. I wasn't really holding anything up. I guess she thought I wasn't being responsible. She blurted out something like, "You know, that's probably your problem. You can't follow schedules." Well, my problem was that I did follow schedules. That was part of my problem. I was following everybody's schedule but my own. I was meeting everybody else's needs. I thought that was very cold, a very low blow. Here I'm thinking, "Gee, there's never time for me." But even though it wasn't the greatest experience in the world, I also knew that I wasn't in an emotional state to leave. It kept me from hurting myself. So, it accomplished that purpose.

Keisha, on the other hand, actually enjoyed her experience in the hospital.

It was really good. I felt there was a bond there. The other patients there could understand. I felt more at ease with myself. Now there was something concrete and valid about the feelings that I had. Before, it was like I'm a weirdo, no one else feels this way.

We would do group therapy. Then we would have lunch,

and after lunch we might do art therapy or dance therapy.
They might let us go outside and play volleyball. There were
a lot of things that we did.

Once your symptoms have stabilized, your doctor may suggest a day hospital program, in which you spend all day at the hospital but go home at night. Day hospital activities are similar to those you might participate in while an inpatient, though since people in day hospital programs are recovering from depression and can be more active, there may be more to do. Cognitive therapy groups, art therapy, and off-campus activities (like visiting museums or going out to lunch) are common day hospital activities. Day hospitals are an important part of recovery for many severely depressed people, and most insurance plans (and even Medicaid) will pay for them.

Drug treatment, ECT, and hospitalization may still seem a bit scary to you. Talk about all your fears with your doctor. He or she will be able to answer any questions you may still have about any of these treatments. If you are in psychotherapy, talk to your therapist about your feelings. Joining a support group may also help. Whatever you do, don't let fear keep you from getting all the help you need. Take advantage of all the tools necessary and available to conquer your depression.

11

· · · · · · ·

Sisters Doin' It for Themselves: Self-Help and Prevention

Up to this point, we have spent ten chapters telling you that depression is an illness, one that you can't control, one that must be treated. Now we are going to tell you something that might not seem to make sense. *You can help yourself get through depression.*

No, we are not suddenly changing our minds and suggesting that treatment isn't necessary. It very much is. But there are numerous things you can do to help yourself through a depressive episode. There are also countless things you can do to improve your self-esteem and strengthen your support network when you are not depressed. Some of these are things you already do to make yourself feel better. Others are new suggestions, things you may not have thought of before. The main point is to pay attention to *you:* what brings you down, what gets you up, what helps you out.

Those Three Little Words: I'm Worth It

Most depressed women (and quite a few of those who aren't depressed) have trouble making time for themselves. They don't think they are worth it. There are legitimate reasons why making time for ourselves is hard: we have children, husbands, boyfriends, girlfriends, parents, brothers, and sisters who need our love, attention, and advice. We have jobs and classes. We have shopping and cleaning and cooking to do. And all of this is important.

But neglecting the self is a sure way to exacerbate stress, which, as we know, can trigger depression in people who are vulnerable to it. Neglecting the self also sends a negative message to others in your life. It tells them, "I don't think I'm important. I don't believe my time is valuable. You don't have to, either."

Depression compounds this problem by making it even easier for you to ignore your needs. You feel worthless and hopeless, so why bother? But it is precisely at this time, when you feel your worst, that spending time on yourself is most important. If you can begin to counter your feelings of worthlessness, you may be able to keep your depression from getting out of control.

Six Steps for Self-Help

One of the most upsetting aspects of depression is that it undermines your control of your life. These self-help steps were designed to help you maintain or regain some of that control.

Step 1: Know your personal depression warning signs.
Step 2: Make a "To Do for Me" list.
Step 3: Establish a support circle.
Step 4: Keep a thought journal.
Step 5: Set up a schedule.
Step 6: Know when to get help.

Step One: Know Your Personal Depression Warning Signs
Though there are universal, recognizable symptoms of depression, everyone experiences the illness in her own way. Some

women know they are becoming depressed because they begin to feel sad and cry at the slightest provocation. Others become irritable and withdrawn. Think about the times you were depressed. What was your first inkling that something was wrong? Did you:

- Cry a lot for no reason?
- Become short-tempered with your children, friends, or other family members?
- Stay in bed all day?
- Get tired easily?
- Have trouble concentrating?
- Not want to do anything?
- Ignore your appearance?
- Have insomnia?
- Wake up too early?
- Feel achy?
- Crave certain foods?
- Lose your appetite?
- Think about death?

This list is just to get you started. Think about what you felt when you were depressed. Make a list of those feelings that seem to be red flags warning of an impending depressive episode.

Step Two: Make a "To Do for Me" List
Your "To Do for Me" list should include anything that makes you feel good, or feel good about yourself. Some examples might be:

- Exercising
- Taking long, hot, fragrant baths
- Listening to good music

- Pampering yourself: getting a manicure or pedicure, getting your hair done, getting a facial or a massage
- Going window shopping
- Having lunch or dinner in your favorite restaurant
- Cooking or baking a favorite dish or a dish your partner or children especially like
- Reading a novel
- Going for a long walk
- Renting old movies or going to see new ones
- Meditating
- Praying or going to church
- Doing yoga
- Singing or playing a musical instrument
- Writing poetry or keeping a journal
- Calling old friends
- Sewing
- Playing cards

Again, this is just a list to get you started. Write down anything and everything that makes you feel better.

Step Three: Establish a Support Circle
If you are like most people suffering from depression, you retreat from others when you start to become depressed. Even if you can't physically retreat, those close to you may notice that you pull away or that you don't want to talk or go out. The last thing you may want to do is be around people.

This is why it is important to establish a support circle *before* you experience another depressive episode. Your support circle should be made up of people who understand your depression. They must be willing to be supportive in the way that you need them to be, not in the way they want to be or think is best. This is key. Your support circle is about you and for you.

Setting up your support circle. Make a list of two to four people who you love and trust who you feel could be supportive when you are depressed. Be honest with yourself. Don't put your sister on the list if she doesn't make you feel supported. Your support circle can include family members, friends, counselors or therapists, and even your minister or priest.

Think about how these people can help you when you are depressed. Do you want them to call you from time to time? Do you want them to go out to lunch or to the movies with you? Maybe you'd like to exercise together. Go through your "To Do for Me" list. Decide which of those things you'd like to share with a member or members of your support circle.

Sit down with each of them separately and explain that you would like to be able to rely on them for support when you are depressed. Make sure they understand that depression is an illness and that you are not being lazy, self-indulgent, self-pitying, or self-absorbed when you are depressed. Tell them exactly what you *don't* need to hear when you are depressed (see the box on page 220). Suggest that they read about depression. And be certain that they understand the seriousness of what you are asking. Tell them in no uncertain terms that they may be saving your life by being there for you when you are depressed. Prepare them for the possibility that you might be suicidal. Make sure they understand when you should get professional help. Tell them that they may have to keep medications for you (if you are a suicide risk) or that you may need to stay with them for a while. Being a part of a depressed person's support circle is a big responsibility. Do not be upset if some of the people you ask can't promise to do it all. It might also be helpful to join a depression support group (see below).

Step Four: Keep a Thought Journal
A thought journal is different from the journal you may keep to record your feelings, reflections, and dreams. The purpose of the thought journal is simple: to help you understand and control your negative thoughts.

Buy a notebook or journal. If having a pretty, more expensive journal to write in will help you feel better, then by all means get one. Otherwise, a simple spiral-bound notebook will do. Just make sure it is small enough to carry with you at all times. Every time you have a negative thought about yourself, write it down in your journal. For example, if none of your friends called today, you might think, *My friends don't want to be bothered with me.* Write that thought down in your journal. Then ask yourself, *Is this really true? What might be some other reasons why my friends didn't call today?* Write these down, too. Then make a note of something you can do to change the situation. If your friends didn't call, make a note to call them, and do it. Challenging your negative thoughts in this way can help you begin to understand how they influence your mood, and it will help you overcome them.

Step Five: Set Up a Schedule

Depression can make you feel overwhelmed, as if every little chore will take your last drop of energy. Making a daily schedule when you are depressed can help you determine what you can accomplish and what might be too much to try. And checking things off your schedule can make you feel better because you got something done.

Make a list of all the things you have to do each day. If it isn't essential, don't write it down. Don't clutter your schedule with things you think you should do. Just list the basics. Add a few things that will help brighten your spirits, too. Divide your day up by hours. Plan out what you will do during each hour of your day. Reward yourself by doing something for yourself every time you check something off your list. Keeping occupied (but not overoccupied) will help keep your mind off your depression, and it will make it a little easier to get through your day.

Step Six: Know When to Get Help

Most of all, know when self-help is no longer enough. Some depressed people know it is time to get professional help when they start feeling suicidal. For others, it is when they just can't get out of bed. You may realize you need help when you can't stop crying long enough to have a conversation, or when you've lost your appetite and have begun to lose weight. Figure out your warning signs. Tell the members of your support circle. If you don't have a therapist or doctor, do a little research while you are not depressed and try to find someone who will be able to help you.

HOW TO HELP (AND HOW NOT TO HELP) A DEPRESSED PERSON

Do:

- Encourage the depressed person to get treatment. Black women especially need to feel that it's OK to get treatment for depression, even if that treatment means taking antidepressant drugs.
- Be supportive. If you are part of a depressed woman's support circle, support her in the way she has asked you to. Don't second-guess what she needs. It is not about you.
- Invite the depressed woman out with you. Ask her what's on her "To Do for Me" list. Plan an activity that she would enjoy. If she is just not up to going out, sit with her. Let her know someone cares about her.
- Take all talk about suicide and all suicidal gestures seriously. Be ready to intervene by taking the depressed woman to the emergency room or staying with her if necessary. Tell her you will take her to the hospital if she feels she is a threat to herself.
- Visit her if she's in the hospital.

Do Not:
- Tell a depressed Black woman "Sisters don't have time to be depressed," or "We're too strong to get depressed."
- Tell her to snap out of it. If she could, she would.
- Tell her she would be better off if she didn't think about herself so much.
- Accuse her of being lazy.
- Avoid her and tell her she is too scary or too intense for you to get involved.
- Tell her to get her act together.
- Tell her that she doesn't have anything to be depressed about.
- Pressure her to do things before she's ready.
- Make her feel weak.

Expanding Your Support Circle: Support and Self-Help Groups

Some depressed women may find that they need more support than friends and family members can give them. Perhaps you want to talk to others who are actually living with depression. Sharing your feelings with others who have been there can help you feel understood in a way that talking to those who have not been depressed doesn't. Maybe your friends and family just aren't capable of giving you what you need. If this is the case, a support group or self-help group might be right for you. Some organizations also offer support groups for family members of people living with depression.

Finding a Support Group
There are several local and national organizations that sponsor support groups for people with depression. Depression After

Delivery (for postpartum depression), the Depression and Related Affective Disorders Association (DRADA), and the National Depressive and Manic-Depressive Association (National DMDA) are the best known. Call or write them for a list of support groups in your area. (See chapter 13 for addresses and telephone numbers.) Local hospitals (especially small community hospitals and those affiliated with universities) may also sponsor support groups. Other places to try include women's health centers, community mental health centers, and some churches.

Starting Your Own Support Group
If you've checked it out and discovered that there is no depression support group in your area, you might want to start your own. Or perhaps you would feel more comfortable in a Black women's support group, but no such group exists. Starting a support group can be an empowering experience, and it doesn't have to be difficult.

First, see what help you can get from other sources. The National Depressive and Manic-Depressive Association and the Depression And Related Disorders Association have materials to help you start a support group. DRADA also offers a group leader training program for those interested in starting and leading a depression support group. The National Mental Health Consumer's Self-Help Clearinghouse publishes a training manual for people interested in starting groups. The National Black Women's Health Project and A Circle of Sisters, another Black women's self-help group, may also be able to help you get your group off the ground.

The next task is publicizing your group. If you are affiliated with one of the national organizations, they can refer interested people to you. If not, consider taking out an ad in the local newspaper (you might want to do this even if you are affiliated with a national organization). Many papers have sections that run free community announcements. Don't put your home address or phone number in the ad; instead, rent a box at the local post office or get a voice mail number (voice mail numbers usually cost about ten dollars a month).

You must also decide where your group is going to meet. Places like churches, community centers, and schools are good choices. Don't meet in your home or office, however. It is best to meet in a neutral location.

It may take a while for your group to develop a stable membership. If there are only two of you for the first few months, fine. Two people can certainly help each other. To boost your membership, think about ways you can expand your group. Have an inexpensive flyer printed and ask local doctors and therapists to post it in their offices. Submit an announcement to run during your local TV or radio station's community calendar. As the word spreads, people will join your group.

Support and self-help groups are not group therapy. They do not provide treatment for depression. Their main purpose is to bring together people who share a common experience so that they can learn from and support each other. Support groups can and do help depressed people get better, but not in the same way that therapy does. The combination of therapy and support groups is a powerful one, however. Taking advantage of both gives you two excellent tools to fight your depression.

12

. . . .

Soul Serenade:
Spirituality and Depression

Black people have always turned to God in times of trouble. Without our strong belief that this life is not all there is, we might not be here today. We are humble in the face of the Divine Spirit—whatever we may call it—that always seems to make a way out of no way.

Faith and spirituality are important when things are going well. When we are depressed, however, faith can literally mean the difference between life and death. When asked why she didn't give in to her suicidal impulses, Renee answers confidently, "It's against my religion." Depression can also test faith, however. Though her faith never truly wavered, Renee did wonder if God was trying to punish her with her depression.

> *My family believes in God, and my mother always instilled in us that we should go to church. In church I learned about God and Jesus and how life is a gift. Even though it is hard sometimes, and I feel like I won't survive, I just rely on God. I see God as the only person I can talk to, and I would rely on him every time I was sick. I was just really praying, praying, praying—praying myself to sleep, praying to get through the day.*

However, there were times that I did get angry, because I didn't understand why this was happening to me. I would have outbursts and sometimes get angry at God—and then I would get angry for getting angry at God.

I would get angry at God until I learned more about him. Sometimes things happen to you for a reason—to try to get you to see something that God is trying to tell you.

Celeste echoes this sentiment. Although she certainly would not have wished to be depressed, she feels she learned something very important from the experience: how to surrender.

Everybody makes mistakes, but it's very difficult for me to get out of difficult situations. Like with the marriage, there were signs a long time ago that it wasn't going to work and I couldn't get out of it. It's like I had invested in it and I just wanted to continue to invest in it and hope that there would be a payoff at the end, that it was going to be worth it. It's real hard for me to give up. But in the past year, I realized I've had to surrender. And I've never been one to surrender. I've been a fighter my whole life. Learning to surrender has been quite an ordeal for me. To pull out the white flag and say sometimes you have to surrender to God, surrender to nature, surrender to the universe, and roll with the flow; that certain things aren't going to work. I don't normally work that way. I make things work. I try to force them to work. It's really been a lesson for me that you have to stop it sometimes.

In her book *The Value in The Valley: A Black Woman's Guide Through Life's Dilemmas*, Yoruba priestess and spiritual teacher Iyanla Vanzant writes about the many valuable lessons to be learned while in life's low points, or valleys:

Valleys are purposeful. They open our eyes, strengthen our minds, teach us faith, strength, and patience. . . . Unfortunately, many Black women have become so accustomed to hard times and bad situations that we think that is all life has to offer. In order for a woman to wake up and get the message of a difficult experience, she must realize there is always value in the valley.

Depression is what Vanzant would call a valley experience, and there is always something to be learned from depression. Some women learn the simple lesson that they must pay attention to themselves, that they, too, are important. Others learn that they must leave stressful jobs or toxic relationships to save themselves. Many learn the connections between their life experience and their depression. By getting in touch with the spiritual, they can learn to let go.

Depression Is Not a Punishment from God

Although there is always something useful to be learned from depression, God does not use depression to punish us. It is very easy for us, especially if we are depressed, to point to something we did wrong or something we feel badly about and say, "God is punishing me for that." But depression is not a punishment meted out by an angry God. God does not get back at us through illness. Viewing depression as a curse from on high only makes us feel worse. (What could be worse than having God against you?)

Getting in Touch with Our Spirituality

What does it mean to be spiritual? Does it mean going to church every Sunday? Does it mean praying the rosary? Does it mean meditating? Yes. But spirituality is not religion. It is the simple and profound act of connecting with the universe, of realizing that we are part of something much larger than ourselves. It is finding peace, locating a center, and being still.

Going to church is one way to get in touch with the spiritual. Many Black women, like Renee, find that the faith of their childhood gets them through the roughest of waters. But some of us have lost touch with the religious traditions we were raised in. We may no longer believe in what we were taught as children. This does not mean we can't have a connection to the spiritual. The spiritual is often found outside of church.

Maya finds spiritual sustenance in other people's spirituality and in music.

> *I have gotten into modern-day philosophers. One of my favorite people is motivational speaker Les Brown. Through tough, very tough times, there is the evidence of other people's spirituality that helps support me. There are people I admire a great deal, like Iyanla Vanzant. Her* Acts of Faith *is just wonderful. Every morning there is something new being brought out for that day and I love it.*
>
> *There are certain songs that help you transcend. Sweet Honey in the Rock's music is some of the only music that I can listen to and be assured that I feel great pride in myself as a Black woman. Bob Marley makes a difference. Robert Cray makes a difference. When he is singing a blues song like "A Change Is Gonna Come": "I'm tired of living but I'm too scared to die. I know a change is gonna come"— that makes a difference. It's like you are hearing what is inside you. Someone else out there feels the same way I do . . . if he is singing that, he can feel it, too.*
>
> *I have a tape of Robert Cray singing with Tina Turner. Robert Cray came out on the stage with her and the two of them did "A Change Is Gonna Come" and tore it up. You know Tina can just melt butter down. She gets on that song, talking about she is tired of living, but you knew Tina was*

not singing the song as entertainment. She was talking about an experience. She says "I'm tired of living." And then Robert Cray came in there and said, "I'm tired but I'm too scared to die." Then the two of them together just went right on in there, "But I know a change is gonna come."

If you listen to stuff like this, you know you are not alone. That is very helpful to me. It is a wonderful stress reliever to sit and listen to something like that, something that just brings you to tears and you think, "I didn't know all that was there." It just all comes out and then you feel okay.

Nona also finds strength and solace in music.

When I'm really feeling down, I pull out my old Nina Simone and Billie Holiday records. There's something about Nina's voice; it resonates. It seems to reverberate throughout your body and soul. Billie can sound both tough and fragile, which is often how I feel. I know life got the best of her, but listening to her is cathartic. Even though the story of her life and death is truly tragic, listening to her doesn't make me sad. I feel I can connect with what she's saying, kind of an "I've been there" thing, but I know I don't want to give in to it. Listening to Billie reminds me that I am not alone in this, and that I simply can't give up.

Other ways to get in touch with the spiritual are:

- Meditating
- Singing
- Walking in a park or in the woods
- Painting or drawing
- Writing in your journal
- Volunteering
- Spending time with children

Spirituality is about wholeness and healing. It is about quieting your mind and realizing that this life is bigger than all of us. For the depressed sister, this is a very hard thing to do, but it is also perhaps the greatest lesson one could hope to learn.

This Little Light of Mine: Seven Women Healing with the Spirit

Though each of the women interviewed for this book has, in many ways, been to hell and back, each is a success story. They demonstrate what can happen when we realize that depression is not normal and that we need help. Not one of the women would call her journey to wellness easy, but all of them would agree that staying the course has been worth it.

The path to healing from depression begins with finding the light within yourself that urges you to go on. The light may be dimmed, it may sputter and flicker, but as long as there is life, the light is sustained. Healing begins with recognizing that your life is worth living, that the light within you is unique and valuable. It is the only one like it, and it was created for a reason.

Most of the women in this book reached a point in their depression where they almost hit bottom. Celeste reached it when she stashed pills in her car and wrote a suicide note; Elaine reached it when she drove herself to the woods and took an overdose; Nona reached it when she found herself hanging out of a twelfth-floor window. But something saved each of these women. Something stopped them and made them think, "I don't want to die." They saw the light within themselves, the glow of spirit, and knew they had to hold on. Whether you believe this light is God, or the ancestors, or a spirit guide, or the soul, it is real. Finding, cherishing, and nurturing it keeps us alive, even when it seems as if nothing will ever get better.

Today, with love and support from family and friends, with professional help, and with spirituality, each of the seven women is moving toward health. Maya continues to see her therapist to work through the abuse she suffered as a child and teenager. She still has her low points, but her therapist, Tina Turner, Sweet Honey, Bob Marley, and Robert Cray get her through. Latrice, also in therapy, finds solace and strength in her singing. Keisha takes her medication regularly, and though she struggles with fears about her future, she has found the hope to pursue her dream of going back to school. Nona, in therapy and taking Paxil, has found that the medication allows her to concentrate enough to be able to get through graduate school while working. She no longer spends days in bed, unable to motivate herself enough to take a shower. Elaine has found that a combination of Wellbutrin and lithium has stabilized her moods enough for her to be a regular sitter for her two grandchildren. Celeste has made many difficult changes in her life and feels that therapy has helped her make those tough choices and live with them. And Renee has found that therapy and her life in her church is helping her replace her deep sadness with equanimity and even joy.

As we stated in the beginning of this book, most depressions can be treated, either with therapy, medication, or both. The seven women who shared the stories of their depression with us are no stronger, no weaker, no different than any of us. They show us that any of us can suffer from depressive illness, and that none of us has to. We hope that their courage inspires you. It has certainly inspired us.

13
· · · · · · · ·
Resources

Mental Health/Depression-Related Organizations

American Psychiatric Association
1400 K Street NW
Washington, DC 20005
(202/682-6000)

American Psychological Association
750 First Street NE
Washington, DC 20002
(800/374-2721 or 202/336-5500)

Association of Black Psychologists
PO Box 55999
Washington, DC 20040
(202/722-0808)

Black Psychiatrists of America
2730 Adeline Street
Oakland, CA 94607
(510/465-1800)

National Association of Black Social Workers
8436 W. McNichols Avenue
Detroit, MI 48221
(313/862-6700)

National Association of Social Workers
750 First Street NE, Suite 700
Washington, DC 20002-4241
(800/742-4089 or 202/408-8600)

American Association of Pastoral Counselors
9504A Lee Highway
Fairfax, VA 22031
(703/385-6967)

Depression After Delivery
PO Box 1282
Morrisville, PA 19067
800/944-4PPD or 215/295-3994

Depression After Delivery is a national organization that provides support, information, and referrals to women suffering from postpartum depression. They publish a brochure on postpartum depression and can provide a list of mental health providers specializing in postpartum depression.

Lithium Information Center
Dean Foundation for Health, Research, and Education
8000 Excelsior Drive, Suite 302
Madison, WI 53717-1914
608/836-8070

The Lithium Information Center collects, organizes, and disseminates information about the biomedical uses of lithium and other treatments for manic-depression. The LIC also publishes materials about antidepressants and other treatments for depression.

National Depressive and Manic-Depressive Association
730 North Franklin Street, Suite 501
Chicago, IL 60610-3526
800/82-NDMDA or 312/642-0049

The National DMDA is a not-for-profit organization established to educate patients, families, mental health professionals, physicians, and the general public concerning the nature and management of depression and manic-depression. National DMDA sponsors support groups for patients and families through local chapters across the country. Some of these chapters publish newsletters and have lending libraries. Call the national office for a directory of local chapters.

National Foundation for Depressive Illness, Inc.
PO Box 2257
New York, NY 10116
212/268-4260
Fax: 212/268-4434
Toll-free hot line: 800/248-4344

The National Foundation for Depressive Illness, Inc. (NAFDI) provides information on major depression and other depressive illnesses through distribution of published materials and operation of a toll-free depression information hot line. Services and materials include brochures, a quarterly newsletter, magazine articles on depression, a bibliography of books on depressive illness, and referral lists of doctors and support groups (this is especially helpful; NAFDI will send you a list of doctors and therapists in your area who treat depression).

National Institute of Mental Health
Information Resources and Inquiries Branch
5600 Fishers Lane, Room 7C-02
Rockville, MD 20857
301/443-4513
Fax: 301/443-0008
Mental Health Fax4U: 301/443-5158
E-mail: NIMHPUBS@nih.gov
Depression/Awareness, Recognition, and Treatment (D/ART) Information Toll-Free Number: 800/421-4211

The National Institute of Mental Health, a branch of the National Institutes of Health, is the federal agency that supports research on mental illness and mental health. NIMH also publishes printed materials about depression and other forms of mental illness. You can call, write, or E-mail for their catalog, or, if you have a fax machine, you can call the Mental Health Fax4U line to receive materials by fax.

National Mental Health Association
1021 Prince Street
Alexandria, VA 22314-2971
800/969-NMHA or 703/684-7722

The NMHA offers patient and family support services, public information, educational materials, and community outreach programs. They can also help you locate treatment and support groups in your area.

National Mental Health Consumer's Self-Help Clearinghouse
1211 Chestnut Street, Suite 1000
Philadelphia, PA 19107
800/553-4KEY (4539) or 215/751-9655
Fax: 215/636-6310
E-mail: THEKEY@delphi.com

The National Mental Health Consumer's Self-Help Clearinghouse promotes consumer-run self-help projects throughout the nation. They offer information and technical assistance to patients and families interested in starting or locating self-help and support groups. They also sponsor an annual conference and publish materials on mental illness, treatment, advocacy, and starting self-help groups.

Black Women's Organizations

A Circle of Sisters
405 W. 147th St., New York, NY 10031
212/459-4806

A Circle of Sisters sponsors support groups across the country. They also publish a directory of Black women's support circles, *Conscious Connections.*

The National Black Women's Health Project
1237 Ralph David Abernathy Blvd. SW
Atlanta, GA 30310
800/ASK-BWHP

NBWHP maintains an international network of self-help groups. They can help you start a chapter if there isn't one in your area.

Books

General Reading on Depression
Beyond Prozac: Brain Toxic Lifestyles, Natural Antidotes & New Generation Antidepressants, Michael J. Norden, M.D., Harper-Collins, 1995.
Living with Prozac and Other Selective Serotonin-Reuptake Inhibitors: Personal Accounts of Life on Antidepressants, Debra Elfenbein, Editor, HarperCollins, 1995.
Living with Tricyclic Antidepressants: Personal Accounts of Life on

Toframil (Imipramine, Pamelor), Debra Elfenbein, Editor, HarperCollins, 1995.

On the Edge of Darkness: Conversations About Conquering Depression, Kathy Cronkite, Doubleday, 1994.

Overcoming Depression, Demitri F. Papolos, M.D., and Janice Papolos, HarperCollins, 1994.

The Depression Workbook, Mary Ellen Copeland, M.S., with contributions by Matthew McKay, Ph.D., New Harbinger Publications, 1992.

The Good News About Depression: Breakthrough Medical Treatments That Can Work for You, Mark S. Gold, M.D., Bantam, 1995.

This Isn't What I Expected: Recognizing and Recovering from Depression and Anxiety After Childbirth, Karen R. Kleiman, M.S.W., and Valerie D. Raskin, M.D., Bantam, 1994.

Undercurrents: A Therapist's Reckoning with Her Own Depression, Martha Manning, HarperSanFrancisco, 1994. (Includes an excellent description of treatment with ECT.)

What to Do When Someone You Love Is Depressed, Mitch Golant, Ph.D., and Susan K. Golant, Villard, 1997.

You Can Feel Good Again: Common-Sense Therapy for Releasing Depression and Changing Your Life, Richard Carlson, Ph.D., Dutton, 1993.

You Mean I Don't Have to Feel This Way? New Help for Depression, Anxiety, and Addiction, Colette Dowling, Scribner, 1991.

Black Women's Health and Well-Being

Body and Soul: The Black Women's Guide to Physical Health and Emotional Well-Being, Linda Villarosa, Editor, HarperPerennial, 1994.

The Black Women's Health Book: Speaking for Ourselves, Evelyn C. White, Editor, Seal Press, 1990.

Girlfriend to Girlfriend: Everyday Wisdom and Affirmations from the Sister Circle, Julia A. Boyd, Dutton, 1995.

In the Company of My Sisters: Black Women and Self-Esteem, Julia A. Boyd, Dutton, 1993.

Racism and Discrimination

The Rage of a Privileged Class, Ellis Cose, HarperCollins, 1993

Two Nations: Black and White, Separate, Hostile, Unequal, Andrew Hacker, Scribners, 1992.

When and Where I Enter: The Impact of Black Women on Race and Sex in America, Paula Giddings, Bantam, 1985.

Women, Race, & Class, Angela Y. Davis, Vintage, 1983.

Relationships

Black and Single: Meeting and Choosing a Partner Who's Right for You, Larry E. Davis, The Noble Press, 1993.

Embracing the Fire: Sisters Talk About Sex and Relationships, Julia A. Boyd, Dutton, 1997.

Friends, Lovers, and Soul Mates: A Guide to Better Relationships Between Black Men and Black Women, Derek and Darlene Hopson, Simon & Schuster, 1994.

Love Lessons: A Guide to Transforming Relationships, Brenda Wade and Brenda Lane Richardson, Amistad Press, 1993.

The Best Kind of Loving: A Black Woman's Guide to Finding Intimacy, Dr. Gwendolyn Goldsby Grant, HarperCollins, 1995.

Wild Women Don't Wear No Blues: Black Women Writers on Love, Men, and Sex, Marita Golden, Doubleday, 1993.

Abuse

Chain, Chain, Change: For Black Women Dealing with Physical and Emotional Abuse, Evelyn C. White, Seal Press, 1985.

Crossing the Boundary: Black Women Survive Incest, Melba Wilson, Seal Press, 1994.

Spirituality

Acts of Faith: Daily Meditations for People of Color, Iyanla Vanzant, Simon & Schuster, 1993.

Black Pearls: Daily Meditations, Affirmations, and Inspirations for African-Americans, Eric V. Copage, Quill, 1993.

Faith in the Valley: Lessons for Women on the Journey Toward Peace, Iyanla Vanzant, Fireside, 1996.

Interiors: A Black Woman's Healing . . . in Progress, Iyanla Vanzant, Writers and Readers, 1995.

In the Spirit: The Inspirational Writings of Susan L. Taylor, Susan L. Taylor, Amistad Press, 1993.

My Soul Is a Witness: African-American Women's Spirituality, Gloria Wade-Gayles, Editor, Beacon, 1995.

Sisters of the Yam: Black Women and Self-Recovery, bell hooks, South End Press, 1993.

Tapping the Power Within: A Path to Self-Empowerment for Black Women, Iyanla Vanzant, Writers and Readers Publishers, 1992.

The Value in the Valley: A Black Woman's Guide Through Life's Dilemmas, Iyanla Vanzant, Simon & Schuster, 1995.

Internet Resources

News Groups:
alt.support.depression
alt.support.depression.manic
soc.support.depression.crisis
soc.support.depression.family
soc.support.depression.misc
soc.support.depression.seasonal
soc.support.depression.treatment

World Wide Web:
www.mentalhealth.com (The Internet Mental Health Page)
www.cmhc.com (Mental Health Net)
libertynet.org (Directory of mental health association information and referral services)

OTHER BOOKS OF INTEREST